The
MAGIC MINDSET

The MAGIC MINDSET

HOW TO FIND YOUR HAPPY PLACE

PREETI SHENOY

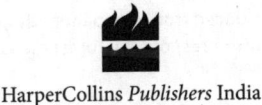

HarperCollins *Publishers* India

First published in India by
HarperCollins *Publishers* 2021
A-75, Sector 57, Noida, Uttar Pradesh 201301, India
www.harpercollins.co.in

2 4 6 8 10 9 7 5 3 1

Copyright © Preeti Shenoy 2021

P-ISBN: 978-93-5422-772-1
E-ISBN: 978-93-5422-773-8

The views and opinions expressed in this book are the author's
own and the facts are as reported by her, and the publishers are not
in any way liable for the same.

Preeti Shenoy asserts the moral right
to be identified as the author of this work.

All rights reserved. No part of this publication may be reproduced,
stored in a retrieval system, or transmitted, in any form or by any means,
electronic, mechanical, photocopying, recording or otherwise,
without the prior permission of the publishers.

Typeset in 11/14 Minion Pro at
Manipal Technologies Limited, Manipal

Printed and bound at
Thomson Press (India) Ltd

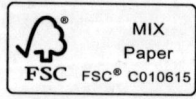

This book is produced from independently certified FSC® paper
to ensure responsible forest management.

For my father, K.V. J. Kamath, the epitome of positivity
My mother, Priya, the epitome of strength
My son, Atul, the epitome of kindness

Contents

Introduction 1

PART 1
Understanding the Magic Mindset

1. The Trouble with Positivity 9
2. External Circumstances and Our Mindset 18
3. The Magic Mindset Can Alter Reality 25

PART 2
Practising the Magic Mindset

4. The Cornerstones of a Quality Life 37
5. Magic Mindset for Money 41
6. Magic Mindset for Relationships 65
7. Magic Mindset for Good Health 87

PART 3
Sustaining the Magic Mindset: Fight the Drains

8.	Magic Mindset and Awareness	115
9.	The Magic Mindset for Situations Beyond Control	118
10.	Magic Mindset for Haunting Memories	141
11.	Magic Mindset for Exams and Interviews	156
12.	Magic Mindset for Reconciling with Other People's Actions	167
13.	The Magic Mindset for Saying No	182
14.	The Magic Mindset for Social Media	191

PART 4
Fun with the Magic Mindset!
A 14-Day Activity Challenge to Help You Start Your Journey into the Magic Mindset

15.	The 14-Day Challenge	203
	Acknowledgements	221
	About the Author	223

Introduction

On 31 December 2019, I went out for a coffee with my daughter. I was happy that she was in India and with me for the new year. We clicked selfies, shared them on social media and wished each other a 'Happy New Year'. We were hopeful and optimistic, looking for a new beginning, a fresh start. Even for the most cynical among us, the start of something is always exciting. It feels like a blank canvas on which we are free to paint as we please.

When we wished each other joy, health, happiness, prosperity for the next year, we sincerely believed it would be better than the last. The year 2020 was special—not only was it a brand new year but also a brand new decade.

Little did we know it would turn out to be one of the worst we'd ever faced.

I had grand plans, like many of us. My thirteenth book was to be launched, and tours had already been planned. The marketing strategy was in place. Months of effort that went into writing would now culminate in a physical book—one of the highlights of a writer's life.

In March 2020—when the pandemic had only just reared its ugly head and we had no idea what lay in store—I was in Mumbai for the cover launch of my book. There was uncertainty in the air, but the magnitude of what was to come had not sunk in yet. My book event was cancelled, and I barely managed to make it back home to Bengaluru. I did not know it then, but it would be at least five more months before I could step out of my residential complex.

On the personal front, I had planned to be in Singapore in August 2020 to watch my children graduate. As the lockdowns kept getting extended, I began to lose all hope of seeing my children any time soon. After several months of uncertainty, my son and my daughter managed to move countries during the pandemic on special evacuation flights, and successfully completed the mandated quarantine. I think I greyed more in fifteen days than I have done in fifteen years.

Eventually, my book launch was organized online. My children's graduation ceremony was online. They happened, and we were glad, but they just didn't feel the same.

A writer's job is a solitary one. Even before the pandemic struck, my work did not involve going out or meeting other people. I stay at home, and I let my imagination soar. My office is inside my head. And yet, the pandemic affected me badly. One cannot be immune to what is happening around them. For months, I was in such shock that I couldn't work on any fiction.

The world had turned upside down. As I type this, the dreaded COVID-19 has taken the lives of over 2.78 million people worldwide. It has caused losses amounting to billions of dollars. Today, we are in a strange situation, forced to co-exist with fear, uncertainty and a general bleakness hanging in the air. Though vaccines are now out, there's not a single person I know who believes this will pass and things will return to 'normal'. The idea persists that this is the new normal and that we must make peace with it. Many people told me that during the lockdown, they felt claustrophobic, as their apartments had no balconies. They craved fresh air. They wanted to go to the gym. They fell into depression, isolated and cooped up. They felt they had nothing to look forward to in life.

When the first lockdown was announced in India, I started a series of blog posts called '21 Days of Positivity'. Every day, I would write a new blog post, which people could read in their inbox, free of cost, if they subscribed. As the lockdowns kept getting extended, I continued posting on my Instagram account simple things that give joy. To my surprise, I began receiving hundreds of messages of gratitude and thanks, telling me that my posts were the only things helping people get through the day, urging me to write more such posts. It was overwhelming to think that whatever I shared was having an impact on people's lives.

A lot of people also wrote to me asking if it's truly possible to be happy all the time? They said I made it seem easy. How does one be positive when the reality is harsh? Does one take a Pollyannaish approach, pretending that the situation does not exist? Do we ignore the terrible statistics of deaths and the crippling economic growth that stare at us everywhere we look? How do we manage it?

When I started responding to the queries, the replies became longer and longer. Many asked me to put them up so they could refer to it whenever they felt the need for a 'pick-me-up'. I began talking to people, asking them what they found most difficult about being hopeful. As they opened up to me, I discovered I had a lot of suggestions and tips to offer. After all, I had some experience in facing grief.

A few years back, I had faced the biggest loss of my life, a tragedy from which I thought I would never recover. But eventually, I did. I also inadvertently discovered a precious skill—that we can indeed change our mindset and cope with anything that life throws at us. I call this the 'magic mindset'.

The magic mindset consists of a set of principles for every area of life, designed to help us shift our perspective from hopelessness to hope, from despondency to joy, from cynicism to belief—a belief that change is coming, and things are not as bad as they seem. If we view our problems through the lens of the magic mindset, they don't seem that big or daunting.

While the principles capture the general idea, what is hard is to put those principles to practise. In this book, I have offered practical steps we can take in situations that trouble us, so that we feel more in control. I have also come up with exercises within each chapter, which can help us define the exact problem facing us.

Often when we think of a problem we are facing, our thoughts are jumbled. They go on in a loop, binding us, rendering us helpless as we get caught in a never-ending cycle of stress, stemming from inaction, simply because we feel helpless. We do not think clearly when we are *within* the situation.

The questions in this book require that we contemplate a bit before answering. There are no right or wrong answers. One person's reality and journey can be completely different from another's. I encourage doing every exercise as it comes up, before reading further. At the end of the book, there is a

'14-Day Magic Mindset Challenge' to gently nudge us towards the magic mindset journey.

This book does not have to be read in any particular order. For instance, if you feel you are happy about most things but your relationships could do with a little help, turn to that section. But whatever section you choose to read, the book will not help if you read it like a novel and rush through it! It requires active participation, and whatever I outline in these pages should be practised.

I have followed all of it myself and shared everything that helped me. I have also included anecdotes from which we can all be inspired. I have shared personal stories from my life too.

You can keep returning to the exercises whenever you feel the need for it. Your answers might be different based on your changing circumstances and your mindset at that point in your life. Keep practising and be consistent. If you do, I assure you that you'll begin to see a change in your outlook.

It is my sincere wish that whatever I have shared here helps you on your journey towards the magic mindset and, brings you joy and hope. This mindset has helped me achieve my dreams, and I hope that it helps you achieve all your dreams too.

Thank you very much for picking up this book.

Love, light and healing,
Preeti Shenoy
April 2021

PART 1

Understanding the Magic Mindset

1

The Trouble with Positivity

Sometimes the questions are complicated and the answers are simple.

—Dr Seuss

IN 2005, I REMEMBER SITTING IN A MULTIPLEX WITH A group of friends, clutching my tummy and laughing helplessly till tears rolled down my eyes, at one of the silliest Hindi films I've watched till date. The movie, *No Entry*, among the biggest hits of that year, starred Anil Kapoor in a comic role. The character that he plays keeps advising his friend to 'be positive', especially when they are both in the kind of trouble from where there seems to be no escape, and they are likely to get thrashed. In exasperation, the friend asks 'Why do you keep saying this? What is this "be positive"?'

'Oh, it's just my blood group,' he replies. 'I will need it when we're beaten up and lying in the hospital.'

Anytime I hear the phrase 'be positive', it takes me back to the movie. The phrase, due to its overuse, especially in today's times, has become hackneyed. When the circumstances are grave, the phrase can almost sound like a joke. We all want to see bad situations in a new, hopeful light. But how do we do that? What if there's really no solution?

This is where the 'magic mindset' helps. While positivity tells us to look at the bright side of things, the magic mindset embraces and accepts that it is not always possible to look at the bright side. Sometimes, things are so bleak that our mind refuses to accept that there can be anything positive about it.

Positivity as People See It

According to the Oxford Dictionary, positivity is a practice of being optimistic in attitude. According to the Cambridge Dictionary, positivity means the quality of having a positive attitude. They state the opposite as 'negativity'.

Since there is a lot of talk about 'being positive', curiosity led me to ask different people what they thought positivity meant. My nineteen-year-old daughter said, 'Positivity means finding the good even in the worst situations.'

When I posted the question on my social media, I got over a hundred responses in a few hours. The answers offered me glimpses into people's world views—a cross-section of their minds, their philosophies, their approach to life and what they believed in.

One definition that stood out was that positivity meant keeping our arms open to embrace everyone, especially ourselves; only then would thoughts not linger longer than required and only then can one understand self-love. If we managed to do this, we could also accept diversity and opinions and thoughts different from ours.

Another respondent said that he wakes up and gets out of bed because of positivity. To him, positivity was hope that the day that lay ahead would be better than the one he had yesterday. Yet another defined positivity as 'Karma'. She believed that whatever we faced daily was because of our Karmas, and she tried to stay calm knowing this too would pass. Another said that positivity is finding an oasis of peace within ourselves, despite all the external circumstances.

Exercise 1

Take a few moments to think about what positivity means to *you*. Please write it down here.

Read the definition that you have written. How does it make you feel? Do you think the phrase is overused? Do you think that it is possible to apply the definition you have written to all situations life throws at you?

The Magic Mindset and Reality

For some people, the very word 'positivity' is an irritant. They believe that positivity lulls us into a false sense of not seeing reality for what it is. How can we be positive about, say, our finances, when the credit card bills have piled and we are broke? How can we say that the world is beautiful when millions in it are dying? How can we be positive if a loved one has been diagnosed with a terminal illness? What if the person who means the most to us is snatched away suddenly?

That is exactly what happened to me when I lost my father, out of the blue, with no warning whatsoever. He was supposed to visit me a week after the day he died. Instead, he leaned back in his chair and passed away, in the middle of a conversation with my mother. And the surprising part? He was absolutely healthy and had no age-related ailments. He used to walk about ten kilometres every day. He had meetings scheduled the next day. He was sixty-five.

Since I was very close to my father, speaking to him almost every day, you can imagine what a massive shock it was. It felt like my world had ended. For a year, I didn't smile, socialize or talk to anyone. My father was one of the most cheerful people I knew, and one of the things he would keep emphasizing was that no matter what happened in our lives, we always have choices. We can choose to see things differently. This is the essence of the 'magic mindset'. It is viewing things differently, looking at them from an angle that we never considered before.

A few years ago, I was studying portraiture in the UK. Our task was to make drawings from real-life models who would pose for a couple of minutes. We would all stand in a semi-circle around the model and draw what we saw. Though we were all looking at the same model, our drawings would all be starkly different. The instructor encouraged us to walk around the model and see how even the slightest movement on our part changed how we viewed them.

Life is like that. Two people faced with the same tragedy will view the event in different ways.

As for me, after my father's death, I found it very hard to view things 'differently'. How could anything change the fact that my father had been snatched away from me? It was so unfair. I was plunged into darkness. I didn't want to wake up in the morning or get out of bed.

To cope with the spiral I was experiencing, I started a blog. I decided that I would focus only on the positive things, no matter how small, that happened to me during that day. There was a lot of sadness in my life, yet I chose to cling on to the tiniest happy thing I could think of. Without knowing or realizing it, I was doing exactly what my father had ingrained in me; I was applying the principles of the *magic mindset*.

The magic mindset helps us view things in a way that is most advantageous to us at the current stage of our life.

In the initial days, no one read my blog. But I was writing because I didn't know what else to do. I missed my father terribly. I couldn't accept that life could change so suddenly. My father believed that we could achieve whatever we set out to, if we were determined enough, and that included happiness. He used to tell me, 'Nobody can make you unhappy without your permission.'

As I learnt to cope with the shock and the numbing grief of his death, I began focusing on what was going right, something my father had always advocated. I had a goal now, a way to fight the inner darkness—focus and write about one single happy thing that I could think of. Some days, even when I felt that I had nothing to write about, I would think hard and find something. As the months went by, the footfall on my blog grew. Though I was writing primarily for myself, my words soothed many. It has been over fourteen years now, and I continue to blog—not daily any more, but regularly.

Changing How We View Our Reality

The bottom line is that even in our darkest moments, when all we feel is overwhelming sadness, we can find *one* good thing and focus on that. It can be something as small as finding a footwear that fits well or watching sunlight filter through the trees.

While the standard idea of 'positivity' leaves no room for any kind of sad feelings, the magic mindset encompasses all kinds of feelings. It does not require us to suppress our feelings of sadness and allows us the space to be unhappy.

The award winning 1997 Italian movie *Life Is Beautiful*, directed by Roberto Benigni, is a fabulous example of what the magic mindset is all about. The movie depicts the heart-wrenching and inspiring story of Guido, a young man living in Italy in 1939. Cheerful, exuberant, a bit of a prankster, Guido falls in love with Dora, who is engaged to a rich but arrogant man. Guido sets up many 'coincidences' to express his interest in Dora, and they eventually elope. They have a son, Joshua, and make their living running a bookstore. During the German invasion, Guido and his family are rounded up by the Nazis and sent to a concentration camp. Guido and Joshua are separated from Dora and sent to a different concentration camp. There, Guido uses his sense of humour and imagination to keep five-year-old Joshua safe from the horrors of the camp.

He tells Joshua that it's all a game and that he has a chance to win a real army battle tank, which Joshua is excited about. He says he will lose points if he cries, if he asks to see his mother, or if he is hungry and asks for a snack. Though there are terrible, unimaginable atrocities being committed, Guido shields Joshua from all of it with his attitude and spirit. Joshua never comes to know that all around him innocent people are being murdered and that his father and mother are probably next. Guido refuses to be anything but hopeful even though he knows that torture and inevitable death await him. He clings to life, exploring his vast imagination and creativity, coming up with 'explanations' to shield his son even in a concentration camp where hopelessness, death and torture are the only certainties. If you haven't watched this movie, do watch it. It is one of the greatest examples of how we can look at things differently and develop the magic mindset. Of course, we cannot all be Guido, but we can certainly draw inspiration from his attitude.

Magic Mindset and Feelings

A grouse that many people have with positivity is that there is such a lot of emphasis on it that it often feels forced. Many of us have also been bombarded with messages like 'look on the bright side' or 'there are people who have it worse than you' and so on. The messages invalidate our feelings of sadness or grief, making it seem as though we are not allowed to feel sad about things—because there's always someone else in the world who has it 'worse'. But positivity is not a switch that can be flipped on at will. Feelings of grief or sadness are real for the person feeling them and cannot be wished away. It is not possible nor is it healthy to suppress all our feelings of sadness and ignore reality.

The magic mindset means accepting sadness and being aware of adverse situations, while taking small steps to get through them.

Life throws at us different experiences. It might take away loved ones, a job or money. But through it all, if we maintain a sense of hope despite the grief that envelops us and if we believe that things will eventually get better, then we have succeeded in cultivating the magic mindset.

The magic mindset teaches us to be patient, allowing the grief and hopelessness to flow through us till it no longer controls our actions. It is segregating what we feel from what we do. It is knowing with a quiet calmness that 'this too shall pass'.

No matter what situation we find ourselves in, we can train our mind to think this way. There are steps we can take, to change the way we think. Our thoughts determine our actions, and by changing our thoughts, we can change our reality. Creating a magic mindset can help us brave life's battles, and this book shows you how to do that.

Exercise 2

Before you begin, think of why you want to change your mindset. What do you hope to achieve?

2

External Circumstances and Our Mindset

If you're reading this ...
Congratulations, you're alive.
If that's not something to smile about,
then I don't know what is.
—Chad Sugg, *Monsters Under Your Head*

A FEW YEARS AGO, I VISITED BHUTAN, A BEAUTIFUL kingdom between China and India, on the eastern edge of the Himalayas, known famously for its happiness index. The landscapes were dramatic, ranging from sub-tropical plains to large mountains and valleys.

After a three-hour slippery and steep trek, with the persistent rain adding to the danger, I sat inside the Paro

Taktsang monastery (popularly called 'The Tiger's Nest'), which hangs off the cliff. A strange sense of peace and calmness enveloped me. It was as though I had stumbled upon a treasure inside me. I never knew such euphoric calmness could be experienced by doing nothing but simply being present. Nothing existed but that moment when I closed my eyes standing before the larger-than-life figure of Padma Sambhava. I spent a few minutes in exhilaration and absolute bliss—an almost Nirvana-like state.

I travelled to many places in Bhutan and visited many monasteries. I loved the quaint cafes, the bookstores in Thimpu and the absence of traffic lights on the roads. Anywhere I went, there was a feeling of peace and calm in the air. Almost every person I met had a wise saying or a quote for me. I saw unbridled joy, hope and acceptance. Simplicity was a part of life in Bhutan, and I naturally fell in love with the place. I dreamt of relocating there; I would be happy, forever, in this serene country. I would rent a pretty little cottage by the hills. I would stroll down an idyllic road, dreaming up the plots for my novels and writing in bliss. I wondered if it was possible for anyone to feel negative in such a place.

Later that day, we stopped at an old cafe, overlooking the deodar and pine trees at the foothills of the mountains. We met a European man who had been in Bhutan for a few years and ran a de-addiction centre for youth. Despite everything that the country offered, there were still people falling into addictions, trying to escape their demons. I was stunned. Depression, addiction and other harsh shocks of life weren't something I associated with Bhutan. I was perhaps, naively, viewing Bhutan through rose-tinted tourist glasses.

It made me think deeply about the big role our external circumstances play in how we feel inside. But can we seek peace within ourselves?

We often seek an escape from our problems by 'going on a vacation'. Popular culture leads us to believe that by 'taking a break' from our daily life, we will come back refreshed, better equipped to deal with our stressors. I might have been doing the same with my vacation in Bhutan. But vacations are just that—mini-breaks. They do not magically make our problems disappear. No matter where we go, our problems will accompany us unless we develop a mechanism to cope— the magic mindset.

Breaks are necessary, but we simply cannot take a vacation from life.

Using Our Choices to Develop the Magic Mindset

The same day, when we stopped at a monastery on the banks of River Paro, I came across a famous Buddhist painting called The *Wheel of Life* or the *Bhavachakra* painted outside almost every Tibetan Buddhist temple. It shows the fierce figure of Yama, the god of death, holding a wheel with different divisions. These divisions portray the various realms. Our guide explained to us that Buddhism has six realms in the 'wheel of life'. Things such as addiction and craving fall into the realm of 'hungry ghosts'. No matter how much we ate or drank, our cravings would never be satisfied in this realm. But if we accumulated good Karma by doing good deeds, we would have a chance to transmigrate into other realms. We control our life's path through our actions, which in turn are shaped by our thoughts.

The more I studied the various elements of this painting, the more the painting began to speak to me. Buddhist teaching is founded on compassion, kindness, tolerance and calmness, which lead to peace and positivity. Thus, in the painting Buddha points to the path one can take for liberation from these realms.

We can change our lives by cultivating the right mindset to help us view our problems in a new and helpful light. My father was a great believer in the idea that our thoughts shape our life. Though his job was extremely stressful, we rarely saw him get angry with people. He worked at an oil corporation and was in charge of the entire Kerala region for the distribution of LPG. He had to deal with hundreds of calls from distributors, ministers, government officials, media and many other people whenever there was a supply shortage. When I asked him how he managed to remain so calm even when the people at the other end were agitated, he narrated to me a story about Buddha. It has remained with me ever since.

When the Buddha was walking through a village, an angry man approached him and started yelling. The Buddha stayed calm and did not get affected by the man's words. The man got angrier and abused the Buddha.

The Buddha asked him, 'Tell me, if you bring me a gift and I do not accept it, who does the gift remain with?'

The man was taken aback for a second at this strange question. He thought for a few seconds and said, 'It will remain with me.'

'Well, it is the same with anger. If I do not accept it, it stays with you.'

When my father told me the story, I replied, 'But he could do it because he was the Buddha.' My father replied, 'He wasn't born the Buddha. He was born as Gautama and *became* the Buddha through meditation.'

My father's words had a deep impact on my thinking. We do have choices, no matter our circumstances; we are free to choose how we want to live. We can continue like we always have, repeating patterns that keep us in our comfort zones, performing the same actions over and over, coming back to our beds at the end of a long working day, and then doing it all over again the next day. Or we could choose to live consciously and try to grow, regardless of the external reality.

Choosing the Magic Mindset against All Odds

One of the best books I have ever read on self-growth is Victor Frankl's *Man's Search for Meaning*. Frankl was a leading psychologist in Vienna when he was arrested for being a Jew during the Nazi regime. He survived the Holocaust, and he used his experiences to write the book. Even in the grimmest of circumstances, Frankl found that it is possible to hold on to positivity and hope.

Frankl says, 'When we are no longer able to change a situation, we are challenged to change ourselves.' He talks about how everything can be taken from a person, including their freedom, but the one thing that can never be taken away is their mindset or attitude. He writes about finding a purpose to hold on to, and then immersing oneself in imagining the outcome, that gives us the strength to go on.

The Buddha had the mindset of calmness and acceptance. Viktor Frankl had the mindset of hope. On the face of it, the two are not alike, but they have one thing in common—a focus on something outside their immediate surroundings. They both turned inwards and tapped into the reservoir of strength, and this is something we all possess.

I have met many people in my life whose circumstances and realities are so dark that one would imagine it would seem impossible for them to be happy. Yet, such people are some of the most content people I know.

Many years ago, in McLeod Ganj, I came across a cloth scroll that had a quote by the Dalai Lama:

The True Meaning of Life

We are visitors on this planet. We're here for ninety or one hundred years at the very most. During that period, we must try to do something good, something useful with our lives. If you contribute to other people's happiness, you will find the true goal, the true meaning of life.

—His Holiness the 14th Dalai Lama

Today, the cloth scroll hangs in my bedroom, reminding me that every second we live on earth can be spent meaningfully, as long as we make conscious choices that are in alignment with our personal values.

By activating our magic mindset, we become more pleasant to be around. It is like donning a 'happy hat'. We add value to other people's lives and enhance our own feelings of well-being by looking at our problems differently.

This mindset is something we can all achieve if we choose to do so consciously. Just like we go to the gym and lift weights to train our bodies, we can train our minds. The magic mindset can change reality—and all we need to do is to believe that a different way of thinking is indeed possible.

3

The Magic Mindset Can Alter Reality

You have brains in your head. You have feet in your shoes. You can steer yourself in any direction you choose. You're on your own. And you know what you know. And YOU are the one who'll decide where to go ...

—Dr Seuss, *Oh the Places You Will Go!*

WHEN I ASKED PEOPLE TO DEFINE WHAT POSITIVITY meant to them, not all the answers I received were optimistic. Some felt that it was just not possible to have a 'positive mindset'. If your definition of positivity in Exercise 1 contains some amount of hopelessness, you are not alone. Many felt it was not possible to suspend reality and that positivity asks us to do just that. Another respondent said, 'I am this way, why should I be positive?'

Why Should We Develop an Attitude of Optimism?

It's a good question. Why *should* we be positive? Why can't we live without bothering about whether we are positive or negative or neutral?

Well, almost all research[1] finds that being optimistic has many benefits. These include:

- Increased lifespan
- Better physical well-being
- Lower chances of depression
- Better cardiovascular health
- Better coping skills during stress
- Better interpersonal relationships
- Higher level of performance at work
- Increase in popularity amongst peers
- Higher chances of success in the chosen field.

All this is to say that our mindsets *can* change our reality. The human mind has incredible potential—so much so that it can affect our physical well-being. A tremendous amount of research[2] has been done to understand the functioning of the human mind, and the things the brain has been found capable of achieving are astounding.

---

1   Mayo Clinic and Verywell Mind, 'The Stillness Project'.

2   Dr Rajiv Jhangiani, Dr Hammond Tarry, *Psychology Today,* 'Principles of Social Psychology' (International Edition).

Re-tuning Our Mindset

In 1981, Harvard psychologist Ellen Langer conducted a social experiment.[3] She wanted to test if we could turn back the clock psychologically, and if so, whether it would result in physical changes. She decided to investigate the impact our thoughts and beliefs have on our health, specifically, the ageing process.

As a part of the study, Langer chose eight men in their late seventies. They were invited to live in a residential retreat for seven days. Everything was recreated to make it feel like it was the year 1959, the period when these men were in the prime of their youth. They were all asked to pretend that was the era they were living in. The home had no mirrors. The television was black and white. All the shows that were being played were of that period. The radio played songs of Perry Como and Jack Benny who were popular at that time. Every single object in the home was from that era. Essentially, the men were encapsulated in the past.

When the participants arrived, they went through various tests that measured their mental and physical function. Their memory, cognitive ability, hearing, vision, flexibility … everything was recorded and documented. Twice a day, researchers discussed topics that were important in that era—whether the US needed bomb shelters to defend against a possible Soviet attack, Fidel Castro's advances in Cuba, etc. The men were asked to take part in this make-believe game and pretend it was real. They spoke in the present tense, living this recreated 'reality'.

---

3 The *Harvard Gazette*.

At the end of the experiment, all the men were tested on the same parameters they were tested on upon arrival. The improvements were dramatic, and the results were astounding. Langer noticed a significant improvement in physical strength, hearing, vision, IQ, posture and memory as well as an increase in their overall sense of well-being. The intelligence score was significantly higher for 63 per cent of the participants. The man who had been in a wheelchair when he came in, walked out with a cane. The men who looked frail and weak were playing football on the lawn!

Ellen Langer says, 'Whatever you put in the mind, you also put in the body.' She concluded that our mindset has a much greater impact on our health and ageing than we believe. By extension, changing our mindset *can* change our overall feeling of well-being.

How Mindset Can Work Magic: Living Proofs

Graham Miles and the Locked-in Syndrome

A few years back, when I was living in the UK, I came across the story of Graham Miles in the news. Graham, a father of two, was driving home from work when he suddenly suffered from a brain stem stroke. He slipped into a coma and when he woke up two days later in the hospital, he was completely paralysed from head to toe. The only thing he could move were his eyes. The Doctors called it 'Locked-in Syndrome', a condition in which a person is awake and completely aware of everything, but cannot move or communicate verbally as all voluntary muscles, except the eyes, become paralysed. Individuals suffering from this syndrome even lack coordination between breathing and voice, which restricts them from producing voluntary sounds. Can you imagine the helplessness that someone with Locked-in Syndrome must feel?

Doctors predicted that Graham would never recover, and he would be a prisoner in his body for the rest of his life. Most people with this condition die within a few months and the rest regain only a very small amount of movement.

But Graham was determined to prove the doctors wrong. A few months later, he left the medics utterly bewildered by his remarkable recovery when he took his first few faltering steps. The *Daily Mail* quoted Graham as saying, 'The only thing I could move was my eyelids. Those first few weeks were very strange. I didn't feel any panic or despair, which the doctors said was because the brain produces a mild sensation of euphoria to stop people from going into shock. I remember being puzzled that I felt so calm. The doctors said there was a massive blood clot at the base of my brain and all the nerve endings had died. The junction between my brain and the rest of my body was completely destroyed and the neurologist said I'd never recover.'

Graham said that initially all he did was breathe. He concentrated on that and discovered that in order to breathe effectively, he had to focus on his diaphragm. He did that for two months. Then he started getting a tiny amount of movement in his face. He could utter a word very feebly but could not string sentences together. Still, he kept at it. Then he slowly started trying to concentrate on his big toe, trying to make it move. He closed his eyes and kept visualizing and willing it to move. After about three months, there was a slight, a very tiny movement. He went on to concentrate on other parts of the body.

The doctors have no good medical explanation for what Graham has managed to achieve. He now lives independently and has even taken up motor racing as a hobby. Graham believes that he overcame this devastating condition only by deeply believing that he could. It was his mindset that worked the magic. He is convinced that there is a lot we do not know about what our brains are capable of.

Graham's story inspires, and it reinforces how the magic mindset can overcome what appear to be insurmountable obstacles.

Alison Williams: Transcending Diseases

On NPR's podcast *Invisibilia*, I came across the story of a sixty-eight-year-old Scottish woman, Joy Milne, a retired nurse. She astounded the medical profession with her unusual ability to *smell* Parkinson's disease. Ten years earlier, when her husband (a doctor) was diagnosed with Parkinson's, Joy could 'smell' it on him, though at that time she wasn't aware of what it was.

Joy now works with doctors, helping them 'sniff' out Parkinson's even when there are no medical symptoms, which show up only in the later stages. Parkinson's has many stages. Stage 1 is the onset, when the patient has mild symptoms such as tremors. By Stage 5, patients are no longer able to live alone.

In the course of her work, Joy met Alison Williams, who was sixty-three. Alison had noticed that when she walked in the snow with her husband, his footprints were firm, but hers had a scuff mark, which she chalked up to bad boots. Later, she would become confused about where she was. She consulted a doctor, who diagnosed her with Parkinson's. The diagnosis left Alison feeling helpless and frustrated even in her daily chores. As years passed, everything about Alison slowed down.

This was when Joy entered her life.

Joy says when she first met Alison, she liked her instantly. She was hunched and shuffling, and her voice was so quiet that she had to strain to hear what Alison was saying. After Joy and Alison met and talked, Alison decided she had had enough. She would continue to take the prescribed medications, but she no longer wanted to give in to the feeling of being 'handicapped' and 'trapped'. She simply stopped acknowledging the disease. She refused to worry about what her future would hold and squashed her worst fears. She decided instead to focus on the quality of her life and to do all the things she badly wanted to. She started taking classes she enjoyed: Mature Latin Movers (a dance class), tai chi with weapons and Japanese drumming!

After eleven months of these classes, when Alison met Joy, she was no longer hunched and shuffling. She seemed like a completely different person. And the biggest surprise? Joy couldn't smell the Parkinson's any more—Alison had managed to bring her Parkinson's down from a late Stage 3 to a Stage 1. Joy told Alison that she had no idea what she was doing, but to continue doing it.

Alison said that by changing her mindset, she shifted her focus from the outcome, or on the possibility of a cure that may not come. Instead, she focused on living her life the best she could and, in doing so, succeeded remarkably in reversing the effects of Parkinson's!

Defying Age: The Weightlifting Granny

During the lockdown, the video of an eighty-two-year-old granny, Kiran Bai, went viral.[4] She works out by lifting weights. Her workouts are designed by her grandson Chirag Chordia, who is a trainer. He designed her exercise routine based on what she wanted to achieve. Kiran Bai wanted her joint pains to go away and wanted to be independent.

After six months of persistent training, she saw remarkable results. In the video posted by Humans of Bombay, we can see how the now eighty-three-year-old granny has transformed her life. She is seen pushing away a sofa with her legs, with perfect ease and the stance of a regular gym goer. Her joint pains have vanished.

Magic Mindset: Achieving the Seemingly Impossible

In all these cases the participants achieved something that was considered 'impossible', or in any case, highly unlikely. They did this by choosing to look beyond their present condition or some far-off 'end goal'. They focused only on what they had at the moment. They suspended their belief and self-doubt and just kept at it, taking things one day at a time, doing what had to be done. Slowly and steadily, their reality changed. By taking small actions at a time, and by being consistent, all of us have the power to change our reality if we so desire.

There are many documented medical miracles for which science has no explanation. The human mind is capable of a

---

4   Humans of Bombay (Instagram) and Chirag Chordia (Instagram).

lot more than we assume. Our thoughts have power; ideas have power. People we interact with also have the power to influence our thoughts and thereby our actions.

'Believe and you shall achieve.'

These powerful words have been reiterated many times by many spiritual and personal development teachers. My father too believed that with positive thinking we could achieve anything. He always told me, 'Your mind is the biggest asset you have. Fill it with affirmations, and always believe you can.' It is a piece of advice that has stood me in good stead over the years.

We can change how we feel and how we look at things, without rejecting reality, by changing our mindset and what we choose to focus on.

Exercise 3a

Write down a problem that is overwhelming and consuming you at the moment. Write everything that worries you about it. After you write it down, tell yourself that you have 'released this', and it is no longer in your control.

Exercise 3b

Write down what you can currently control. Affirm that you will focus on this.

PART 2

Practising the Magic Mindset

4
The Cornerstones of a Quality Life

The world is what you make of it, friend. If it doesn't fit, you make alterations.

—Silverado

A FEW YEARS AGO, I VISITED DAKSHINA CHITRA MUSEUM in Muttukadu, near Chennai. I fell in love with this museum, which is like no other I have ever visited. It is a 'living' museum of art, architecture, lifestyle, arts and performing arts. It has a collection of eighteen authentic, historical south Indian homes, and from time to time, there are contextual exhibitions in each house. All these houses had been signed up for demolition by the owners. They were purchased, taken down and reconstructed by artisans from specific regions in the south. Since it is an interactive museum, it also hosts performers, glass blowers, soothsayers, basket weavers and such.

I found myself wandering in awe through a Kerala Syrian Christian house, and a few minutes later, I was transported to Tamil Nadu, walking through a silk weaver's house! In the Tamil Nadu section, I came across an astrologer who could predict a person's future based on cards that his parrot picked. I decided to try it out. To my utter astonishment, the astrologer answered the questions in my mind before I could even utter a single word. He said I have a son and a daughter, and he told me things about my future, my husband's future as well as my children's futures. I wondered how he knew what questions I had wanted to ask. I started chatting with him, and he said that most people have questions that fell into three categories—health, wealth and relationships. He claimed to have read cards for thousands of people and predicted their futures. When I asked him how he knew that I had a son and a daughter, he said the cards had shown him.

Years later, I learnt how to read Tarot cards. As I practised more and more, my accuracy grew. I began reading for close friends and family. The more readings I did, the more I realized that what the astrologer had told me years ago was true. Most people who want a reading from me have questions either about their finances, their health or their relationships. These three are the major areas in all our lives and affect our emotional and physical well-being. Taking complete charge of them ensures that we will lead a more fulfilling life, but rarely is a person in complete control of all three.

Even when everything seems well in all the areas, it is important to not get complacent and check once in a while to ensure things are 'on track'.

Exercise 4a

Give yourself a score on 10 for the three areas in your life, 10 being most satisfied and 1 being least satisfied. 'Relationships' could be with the closest ones in your life—family or friends.

Health:
Finances:
Relationships:

Exercise 4b

Write down your ideal scenario for each of these areas. What would make you give yourself a perfect score? Describe the scenario:

Health:
Finances:
Relationships:

No matter our current fitness level, no matter what we earn right now and no matter how our relationships are at the moment, we can always bring more positivity into these three aspects of our lives and improve them further.

Over the next three chapters, you will discover how.

5

Magic Mindset for Money

Don't think money does everything or you are going to end up doing everything for money.

—Voltaire

WHAT IS THE WORST POSSIBLE SITUATION THAT YOU CAN think of when it comes to finances? For most of us, it is being broke, with zero money in the bank, no place to live and no job. Now imagine going from there to becoming a billionaire business tycoon with a net worth 2.7 billion US dollars.

Sounds impossible? Sounds like a dream? John Paul Dejoria achieved just that.

Principle 1: Always Look Ahead

John was raised by a single mother. At nine, he was selling newspapers and Christmas cards with his older brother, because they were extremely poor. After high school, he joined the Navy for two years, and then got married at the age of nineteen. By the time he was twenty-two, he had a two-and-a-half-year-old son. At the time, John was working as the master of ceremonies at an annual sports vacation recreational vehicle show and had a cheque coming at the end of the week.

One day when he got home, he saw his wife coming down the stairs. She took the car keys from him and left without a word. As he entered his apartment, John saw his toddler son with a note around his neck that said, 'I can't handle being a mom any more. He will be better off with you, good luck.' His wife had left, sweeping the bank accounts clean. She had been planning this for a few months. She had not been paying the rent for months and had kept the money. They were lagging in the payment of several months of rent. Two days later, John was evicted; he was homeless with a toddler son.

John borrowed a car—a 1951 Cadillac—from a friend. The car had a broken water pump, and he had to fill water every four hours for it to keep running. That was how he got going. He started working as a door-to-door encyclopaedia salesman; no salary—only a commission paid on sale. John would visit a hundred houses every day, knowing that most of them would shut the door on his face. He says selling those encyclopaedias was a great lesson that taught him the value of never giving up. He had to have the same level of enthusiasm for the hundredth doorbell he rang that day as he did for the first doorbell.

John was homeless one more time in his life, when he started the Paul Mitchell hair care company along with his hairdresser friend. He needed half a million dollars to start it. He had a good job at the time, lived in a nice house and led a comfortable life. He sold everything and put it into the company. He was all set to start, when the investor backed out at the last minute. John was once again left with nothing but a few dollars in his pocket. He was too proud to tell his mother what had happened or to move back with her. He told her he just needed to borrow a few hundred dollars. John lived in his car; showered in public showers at tennis courts; and went door to door, selling the hair care products.

What stands out in John's story is his resilience. He simply refused to give up. He says it is this mindset that kept him going: he didn't dwell on the past and *only looked ahead*. He just knew that he had to keep going, since lamenting about the past wouldn't put food on the table. *What is the way ahead?* That is all he thought of. John also started the Patron spirits company, which he later sold for 5.8 billion dollars.

John's advice for everyone is that it is possible to get through the most difficult of times as long as we are willing to work hard and put in the effort. Don't sit back, doing nothing. Look for opportunities and grab them.

Principle 2: See with Your Mind, Not with Your Eyes

There are many people in India who have built business empires from scratch, just like John did—out of sheer grit, determination, business acumen and positive thinking. The one story that perhaps all Indians are familiar with is that of Dhirubhai Ambani. Once, he sold fried snacks to make ends meet; today, his Reliance Industries is worth 3.8 trillion rupees!

The lesser-known story of Bhavesh Bhatia is another inspirational one. Bhavesh was born with defective vision. When he was still young, Bhavesh's mother was diagnosed with cancer. Working as a hotel manager, he desperately tried to save money for his mother's treatment but eventually lost her to the disease. His mother had been his pillar of strength, helping him navigate the bullying he faced in school. Even though she wasn't educated, she worked tirelessly to make sure Bhavesh was. By the age of twenty-three, he became completely blind. To Bhavesh, the compounded loss of his vision and his mother felt like the world's greatest injustice. To cope with these devastating losses, Bhavesh turned to one of his strongest interests—creating things with his hands. He attended a training course at National Association for the Blind, Mumbai, and learnt to make candles. Living in a 12 x 15 room, Bhavesh borrowed small amounts of money from his friends. He was able to gather seven thousand rupees and bought twenty kilograms of wax for making candles. He started his industry on a 2x2 corner in that room, with a single candle design. He made them all night long and would sell them from a cart. Whatever profit he made, he invested into buying more wax and making more candles. Today, Sunrise Candles has over 9,700 designs. The twenty kilograms of wax he started with has grown to two hundred tonnes! Bhavesh's company is now a multi-crore business with clients all over the world, and it has a dedicated team of 250 employees—all visually impaired. Bhavesh is very proud of this—to be able to help his employees become financially independent. Bhavesh says that if you can't see with your eyes, that is okay. But if you can't see with your mind, then you have lost everything. It is important to imagine what can be, instead of what is. Only when you can imagine can you take steps to achieve it.

The threads that unite these stories are grit, persistence, and a positive outlook. We can all take inspiration from these stories.

No matter what your current financial position is, it *is* possible to segregate your worries from your financial situation—no matter how severe or bleak it may sound. The first thing to do is to *accept* the impermanence of money and to believe that it is indeed possible to have a mindset where we can greatly reduce the stress and anxiety that comes from the absence of money.

Does this mean we can ignore reality? What if someone has just lost their job, and has outstanding payments? What if they are worried about meeting EMIs? What if the money in the bank will last only a few months, post which they do not know how they are going to survive? How does one remain positive in such circumstances? Can we shift our mindset from that of 'scarcity and fear' to one of abundance?

I am a great believer in the law of attraction and the power of manifestation. Both these laws state that what we focus on, grows. Thus, if we worry about not having enough money, or keep expressing to others that we never have enough, that is what our reality will eventually be. But if we focus on what we do have and express gratitude for it, it will multiply.

I have personally implemented both principles 1 and 2 in my life, to shape the one I currently live. A few years ago, I began reading Rhonda Byrne's book *The Magic*. At that time, I had never made more than thirty thousand rupees for a speaking assignment. I would receive many opportunities, but the colleges that invited me often cited a lack of budget, and I ended up agreeing to speak if they took care of my travel and accommodation, which they always did. I was tired of speaking at events for free, because it ate away a lot of my working days. I was putting a lot of work into these events, sharing all that I learnt through years of experience, putting my health at risk due to constant travelling, spending time away from my family. The people attending these events were all giving fantastic feedback, and yet, for all my efforts, I wasn't getting paid.

The Magic offers small daily assignments for the reader to follow. One of the assignments was to write what you badly need. I wrote that I wanted to be paid one lakh rupees for a speaking event. It seemed like an impossible ask. However, I decided to write it, as the task of that day demanded it. I then forgot about it and moved on to other tasks.

Nine days later, I got a speaking opportunity like no other, where I shared a stage with international stars. And I was paid two and a half lakhs for it! I was astounded at how quickly my wish had manifested into reality. Soon after this incident, I shared it with many of my closest friends. I urged them to buy that book and follow everything written. Unfortunately, since the tasks demand dedication for twenty-eight days, and you have to go back three days and repeat the task if you miss a single day, many of them didn't do it. For the brief period that they did it, they reported feeling less worried. Most of my friends who did the tasks expected something to 'materialize immediately' and gave up when it didn't.

Principle 3: Want It Badly and Believe It Is Coming

For the law of attraction to work for you, you need two things:
1. Whatever you write down must be what you need *very badly*. It must be what you truly wish to attract. You should feel it deeply.

2. You must believe that it *is* coming.

You should also be willing to accept that if it was not given to you, it means that it was not for your highest good and that something even better is coming. I believe completely in the above, and when it comes to money and fame, it has helped me lead a life beyond my wildest dreams, for which I am deeply grateful.

Sceptics would dismiss all of the above. They might argue that it was a mere coincidence that I wrote that amount and only days later the high-paying speaking assignment came my way. But similar incidents have happened far too many times in my life, and I am convinced they are not just coincidences. Those who have never used Law of Attraction before, or who have used it and failed to attract anything, are likely to dismiss these suggestions as preposterous. Money is a tangible, concrete thing. Our bank balance is something that stares us in our faces. How can we not help feeling worried when the situation is stressful?

It may not be possible to feel grateful if you are overburdened with thoughts about what will happen three months or six months from now, when the money runs out. It is impossible to have an abundance mindset in such a situation. It seems like a difficult proposition to *not worry*, especially when you have little money. But it can be achieved. What it requires is a change in mindset.

Just like we do not go to the gym and expect to lift hundred kilograms on day one, we cannot expect to suddenly become worry-free. We need to take small steps, and continuously cultivate optimistic thoughts.

We can't do this by denying reality but by accepting it and then taking practical steps to stop worrying, firmly believing that things *will* change for the better.

Steps to Practice: Use the Magic Mindset to Attract More Money

In this section, I list some of my recommendations that I hope will assist you in seeing the money situation in a different perspective.

1. Take Stock

When we are worried about our financial situation, we must take realistic stock of the situation. When it is in our heads, we tend to magnify problems and make them seem much larger than they are. Worry is like a snowball rolling down the hill. The more we worry, the larger it becomes. One way to tame it is to be rational about it.

If your financial situation is causing you stress, take a piece of paper and write down all the current financial facts. Perhaps you are out of a job, and you are unlikely to get a job for three months (or six months). Perhaps you have suffered terrible losses in your business, and you have been forced to shut down. Perhaps you lack education or hireable skills.

This is the 'problem' that you have defined.

Next, take a look at your bank account and write down the amount of money you currently have. Make sure to include every investment you have made—be it stocks, fixed deposits, mutual funds or anything else that you can think of.

After you do this, write down the value of every single object you own that can potentially be sold. Write down the value of any jewellery that you may own. Write down the value of *all* your assets—your vehicles, your home, everything. Include things that you think you may be able to manage without (for example, television, dining table).

Now, add up everything.

A rather large sum, is it not?

This step of valuating everything you own might seem extreme. But what this exercise does is help you see the value of the things you already own. I am not for a moment suggesting that you sell off any of these things. Instead, this is an exercise in appreciation of what you have already been able to attract. You did all of this without even thinking about it. Now imagine what you could do if you consciously tried.

Exercise 5

Write this affirmation down and stick it where you can see it daily:

The money I need is coming to me. I have been able to create a beautiful life, and I am blessed. Thank you, Universe, for all that I currently have. I am deeply grateful.

Say the affirmation you have written with complete sincerity and emotion. You can modify the words to express what you feel. But it should be a sincere prayer of thanks.

Do this every single day.

Even if you are a student and have no money at all, you can use the above affirmation. Focus on the life you wish to create. Close your eyes and imagine every little detail of your life—let it be like a dream. Say or write the affirmation. Then forget about it and go about your daily business. That's all you have to do.

2. Analyse Expenses and Cut Down

Taking stock is an important first step, but let's now get down to some practical steps we can take to improve our money situation.

c) **Spend less**: If there's one thing the pandemic has taught us, it is that we can do with a lot less than we think we need. With shopping malls closed, no commute to work and no travel, most people tell me that they realize they can still manage. A friend of mine tells me that every weekend, it was a habit to just go to the mall, for want of anything better to do. Each trip she made, she would end up spending about three thousand rupees on average, on things that she didn't actually need. Malls are places designed to make us spend. She says while she has been laid off, her expenditure has drastically reduced as well.

d) **Catch little things**: Most of the time, we aren't aware of the little things that add up. We could start by making a conscious effort to track expenses. Start with things such as the electricity bill and the cell phone plan. Most of us are on a plan that we rarely bother to revise once we have chosen it. The telephone companies keep offering new plans. Examine your current plan against the ones that are now being offered. Sometimes, there are subscriptions to streaming services that we took a long time back, because we wanted to watch a show but later forgot about, and every month the deductions continue. Start catching these 'little' expenses, for they all add up.

e) **Save electricity**: This might seem like common sense, but it is something many of us ignore. CFL or LED lights save a lot of power. Switch off everything not in use. We leave our appliances such as televisions and speakers plugged in, and we don't bother to switch off the main power source. We have also become accustomed to using air conditioners whether or not we need them. If we open our windows and switch on the fans, we can save a lot on electricity. Most of us also leave our geysers switched on for longer than required. While it might be common sense to switch off the gadgets not in use, you will be surprised how many people don't do it! Being mindful about these small things can help us reduce our electricity bills by a lot.

f) **Make a monthly budget**: If we track what we spend on and are a bit more aware while making purchases, it is possible to save more than we think we are capable of. I read about a thirty-day rule for major purchases such as a new phone, a refrigerator or an air conditioner. The rule says that whenever we feel the need to buy something, we should write it down and wait for thirty days. Then, if we still feel we need it, we can buy it. For smaller items, this period can be reduced to twenty-four hours.

g) **Use only cash**: A friend of mine tried a novel method to save money, and it worked. She decided that she would use only cash to purchase things for a month. She decided to withdraw just five thousand rupees and would withdraw more only once that amount had been spent. She was able to cut her expenses by almost 40 per cent! She says since it was inconvenient for her to keep withdrawing cash, she automatically started spending less. Several studies[5] have indicated that people indeed spend more using credit cards. Psychologists attribute this to something called 'coupling'. When we handle cash and spend money, we are painfully aware of how much it costs. Handling the currency notes makes us feel like we are handling a lot of 'real money'. However, when we use a card, there is a gap between when we spend and when we pay, making the cost seem less important. Using only cash is also inconvenient. We need to go to an ATM, withdraw money, and after we pay, we need to get the balance amount, count the notes and check it. With a card, we just swipe and forget about it until the statement comes. Cards also have a 'pay the minimum' option, but if we do the maths, the rate of interest charged on it is exorbitant. Like Will Smith has aptly said, 'We spend money we do not have, on things we do not need, to impress people who do not care.'

h) **Cut your losses**: Many people wait for the 'right time' and the 'right price'. Rafael Badziag, the author of *The Billion Dollar Secret*, interviewed twenty self-made billionaires

---

5 Drazen Prelec, Duncan Simester, 'Psychology of Spending', MIT.

who shared their secrets of success. One of the things that self-made billionaire Peter Hargreaves recommends is to *cut your losses*. He says that he started a venture with an associate and told him that he would give him two years to make it profitable. However, Peter was certain that after six months if he felt the venture didn't look like it would make money, he would have closed them down. Most of the billionaires interviewed in the book say that the best time to act is NOW. The best opportunities to be seized are often disguised around us. If we have idle assets that aren't being used and aren't generating any income, we should sell them off, even if at a lower market value. A friend of mine has a simple principle. She owns an apartment and the rent in that area for an apartment of that size is about sixty thousand a month. My friend rents it out at 10 per cent less than the market value, for fifty-four thousand a month. She has never had a hard time getting a tenant as people jump at the opportunity to rent the place. Her reasoning is that if she waits for the 'right price' to rent it out and the apartment is locked up for three to four months, she loses 2.4 lakhs a year. By renting it immediately at a slightly lesser price, she avoids this loss. I found this to be a smart idea. If we have property that is not being used, it amounts to loss of income. Consider selling it or renting it in ways you never considered before.

3. Try a Different Thing

Losing a job and being unable to find another in the relevant field is often the universe's way of nudging us towards a change.

Many years back, I had a corporate job. I was certain that I wanted a career in management. However, when I gave birth to my son, I couldn't bear the thought of handing over my baby to a day-care and going off to work, so I decided to be a stay-at-home mother. By the time my son was one-and-a-half, I was dying to get back to work. I was tired of having 'no real job'. Yet, I didn't want to be away from my son.

My sister-in-law said that the preschool her child was attending was looking for a teacher's assistant. She asked me if I was interested. I had no experience with children (other than my own son), and I had no teaching qualifications whatsoever. But when I interviewed, the lady who owns the school loved my attitude. I was hired. The best part? I could take my son along with me.

Still, I was scared and the little voice in my head said I might not like it and might fail at it. But I decided to take a chance and give it my best. If I didn't like it, I would have at least explored an option.

It turned out that working at the school was the best experience I ever had. I enjoyed being around the kids—all between the ages of two and four. The teacher I worked for had over twenty years of experience with children. She trained me well. Children are naturally creative, and I discovered I could use my creativity in ways I could have never imagined. I narrated stories, sang rhymes, came up with innovative games and had a whale of a time. My toddler son was happy, and I was *extremely* happy.

Each morning when I opened the gates of the school, there would be an army of small children that poured in yelling in delight, 'Preeti aunty, Preeti aunty!' I had to hug each one of them before I entered the classroom. Their love was so pure, so genuine. What joy!

It is something I would never have experienced in a corporate career. I wasn't making as much money as I would have made in a corporate career, but I was gaining invaluable experience. After a few years, I started my own workshops for children, as I realized that the education system in India does not sufficiently encourage creativity. The workshops were a huge hit.

When we consider doing things we have never done, it leads us down paths we never imagined we could be on. Had I not been open to exploring various options, compromising a bit on the money I made, I would have never started the workshops.

If there's anything that you have always wanted to try, this is the right time. Go for it!

4. Think Creatively

The Better India recently featured the story of N.K. Krishnan Nair, from Aranmaula, a small village located in Kerala. In the centre of the town stands an acre of stunning yellow marigold flowers. It seems like it has popped out of nowhere amidst the pandemic. Krishnan Nair had retired from his job in Libya and decided to settle down in his hometown. He noticed that the land next to his home was rocky and had been lying barren for many years. Krishnan decided to cultivate marigold flowers, since Kerala was experiencing a shortage of these. He gathered information on the soil needed and the best way to go about starting this. He sourced around a thousand marigold saplings from Bangalore and sought advice from farmers who were growing them in Bangalore. Krishnan had to hire JCB machinery to till the soil, and he improved the nutrient quality by adding many organic components. Today, he harvests about fifteen to twenty kilograms of marigold flowers every day, which earns him thirty-five thousand rupees a month. He has now tied up with vendors who collect flowers from this farm in the middle of the city. Krishnan says his little city farm has inspired many to start their own business.

A very enterprising lady I know, a senior citizen, runs a travel agency for fellow senior citizens. Many groups of elderly people have travelled the world along with her. Thanks to her venture, they have visited France, Belgium, Switzerland, Thailand, Malaysia and Dubai to name just a few places. Being a senior citizen herself, she is aware of the problems and discomfort that senior citizens face. Her enterprise is extremely successful, with a lot of people booking months in advance to be with her group. She not only takes care of their comfort during travel but also has arrangements with hotels abroad where they cook food they are accustomed to. After the lockdown put a break on her business, to preserve her sanity, she started a cloud kitchen. Her former tour manager now delivers delicious home-cooked meals she makes. The demand for her food is high, but she has deliberately restricted her clientele because she isn't doing it for the money. She wants to keep herself occupied during the lockdown and help people eat healthy home-cooked food. Today, she is in a position to scale it up by employing more people, but she has chosen not to.

Many people I know have started successful cloud kitchens during the lockdown after being laid off. They consider it a blessing in disguise to have been pushed into this—something they would never have ventured to try had they remained in the safety and comfort of their jobs.

If you have lost your job and have always been wanting to try something new, consider this a blessing in disguise. Do the necessary groundwork and dive in. The best time is now. The best day is today.

5. Create Passive Streams of Income

The average millionaire is estimated to have seven passive streams of income. It doesn't mean that the person has to work seven jobs but that they have created means of earning money in addition to their main income.

Check your area of expertise and watch out for ways in which you can leverage it. For example, if you are interested in gardening, perhaps you can consider starting a garden gift shop as a second source of income. I know someone who holds a regular corporate job. He is interested in bonsais and would previously indulge in it on weekends, as a hobby. Slowly, he also started writing articles about them and began getting paid for it. He started conducting workshops for those who wanted to learn. He began supplying to hotels and nurseries. Ultimately, he became so successful at it that he earns more from his hobby than he does from his corporate job!

Kiran Dembla, who was a housewife, was featured on Humans of Bombay. After her marriage, she was confined to her home. Every morning, she'd wake up and cook for her family and take care of the house. Before she knew, ten years had gone by. She wasn't doing anything she loved. She wanted to do something and started taking music classes for children at home. Still, because she barely left her home, her mental health deteriorated, and she put on twenty-five kilograms. Tired of living this way, she joined a gym. She'd wake up at 5 a.m. to head to the gym so that she could be back at home in time to send the children to school. The gym transformed her life. In seven months, she had lost twenty-four kilos. She became obsessed with getting a six pack and was soon the fittest she had ever been in her life. She achieved all this in eight months. Then, she decided to open a gym herself. She sold her jewellery, rented a flat and converted it into a mini-gym. The Indian Federation of Bodybuilding heard about her and decided to give her an entry into the body-building world championship. Though she faced hardships and had many obligations towards her family, she persisted. She competed in Budapest and won sixth place. She finally decided to live her life and do everything she wanted to do and had missed out on. At forty-five, she is a DJ, a mountaineer and a photographer. She says that the most important thing, however, is that she is the best version of herself.

6. Do More with What Is Already There

My mother lives in Kerala, and she narrated to me the story of a lady who was severely depressed. She had just lost her sister to cancer, for whom she had been the primary caregiver. This lady (let us call her Valsala) had no source of income. The meagre savings that she and her husband had were exhausted as they had spent them on her sister's treatment. Valsala was severely depressed, and they had no money to spend on mental health treatment. Seeing her in this condition, Valsala's father was desperate. To pull her out of her depression, he gifted her a plant and asked her to look after it. Valsala did that. The plant flourished under her care. When it grew, she had to trim it. Instead of throwing away the branches, she planted them in another container and those flourished too. When one of her friends visited her, she liked the plant so much that she offered to buy it. She paid Valsala ten rupees for it. Valsala says that though the amount was small, the hope it gave her was incomparable. She decided to make many more plants. Soon, she had gathered other varieties and started a nursery. Today, Valsala and her husband own a flourishing business with two trucks, which they use to supply plants to many other establishments. It all began with the one thing that Valsala focused on—a single plant that gave birth to a big venture.

If you have a specific skillset, explore the option of creating a class online. If you think you have experience in a certain area, try offering a consultancy. Maybe you love doing up the interiors of a home. Consider doing the makeover for a friend's place, and then share the 'before' and 'after' pictures. Begin with the things you already have that you might be overlooking.

7. Let It Go: Believe and Trust

In the book *The Secret*, Rhonda Byrne says, 'If you are complaining, the Law of Attraction will powerfully bring into your life more situations to complain about.' The Law of Attraction says that whatever we focus on, grows. If we keep worrying and thinking about how little money we have, we are perpetuating in a 'debt situation' unknowingly.

This might seem hard to process at first. If we don't have money, how can we pretend that everything is okay? To pretend we have money would be deluding ourselves.

However, it does become easier with practice. We have to train our mind to focus on the abundance that we are blessed with instead. The universe does not hear the word 'no'. If we say 'I do not want to go broke', the universe is going to hear 'I want to go broke.' Thoughts are powerful and they can shape our attitudes and beliefs. Instead, we could say, 'I want to have enough money to pay for everything I desire, and I am grateful for the amount of money I currently have. Thank you, Universe.'

Use affirmations like the above, which are positive and uplifting. If you are interested to know more about this process, do read *The Secret*, which explains in great detail the way to achieve a change in attitude.

Remember, money is not everything in life.

One of the things that stood out to me in the book by Rafael Badziag is that most billionaires admitted that they have no family life at all. They work long, long hours—probably sixteen to eighteen a day. They are married to their businesses. They are happy because that's what gives them joy. Their work itself is a source of joy for them—not the money they make. Most of them live simple lifestyles. The things that make them happy are not luxury watches and seven-star hotels, but simple things that are accessible to all of us.

In order to change our mindset from that of worry to that of abundance, we have to take small practical steps towards our goals. We also have to remember the impermanence of money and remind ourselves that we can never have enough of it. Man's desires are endless. Our monkey minds delude us, telling us we would be happier with a 'bigger house' and a 'bigger car'. The fact, however, is that once we are there, we would probably crave for something fancier. *The wants are endless.*

On the other hand, what gives lasting peace and joy comes from deep within us. Having money is not the only measure of how rich one is. We must focus on the priceless treasures we already have—whether it is great health or a supportive family or caring friends.

When I was a child, I loved to collect quotations from great philosophers and thinkers. It was the pre-internet era. Access to information at our fingertips, like we have today, was non-existent. Hence, any nugget of wisdom I came across, I wrote down in a little diary, which was my personal book of quotes. I would pore over these quotes and often discuss them with my father. Little did I realize what a powerful impact these words were having on me and how they were shaping my young mind.

One of the quotes I wrote down in that book was this: 'Money will buy a bed but not sleep; books but not brains; food but not appetite; finery but not beauty; a house but not a home; medicine but not health; luxuries but not culture; amusements but not happiness; religion but not salvation—a passport to everywhere but not heaven.'

It remains, to this day, one of my favourite quotes about money.

About twenty-five years back, when I got married, we couldn't afford to buy a car. We would go to company-organized get-togethers in the freezing north Indian winter on my husband's motorbike, while other families would arrive in their cars. We were young, madly in love and we laughed off our situation. When I contracted malaria and was barely conscious, my husband felt terrible that he had to take me on his motorbike to the hospital.

Today, we own two cars, a couple of homes and I am grateful that we are financially well off. However, has our level of happiness changed? Not really. We are just as content as when we got married. The true happiness doesn't depend on our bank balance at all.

George Lorimer said, 'It is good to have money and the things that money can buy, but it is good too, to check up once in a while and make sure you haven't lost the things money can't buy.' While many spiritual gurus and philosophers have expressed the same sentiment in different ways, I can vouch for it as I have lived this truth!

A Malayalam movie I watched, *Trance*, has a scene where the protagonist, who has grown up in dire poverty and who juggles two jobs to make a living, is offered a dream job as an evangelist. He is asked to name his salary. When he hesitates, the guy offering the job keeps raising the amount. The protagonist is astounded when he is offered one lakh, an amount he cannot even picture.

Then, the guy offering him the job raises the amount even higher, going into crores of rupees. He says that man's need is such that no matter how much money we have, we quickly get used to the living standard that it can buy us, and then we want more. This scene struck a chord because it depicted beautifully what I believe in, and what many philosophers and social scientists have reiterated—that the desire for money is insatiable. Seneca summed it up well when he said, 'It is not the man who has too little, but the man who craves more who is poor.'

Many studies have been conducted on winners of lottery tickets[6]. Winning the lottery does make them extremely happy. However, a year later, the level of happiness they feel remains the same as the time before they won the lottery[7].

Whenever we are worried about money, we should follow the above steps and then remind ourselves of three things:

1. No matter what the current situation is and how hopeless it seems, it shall pass.
2. Our happiness needn't depend on our bank balance.
3. No matter how much we make, it will never be 'enough'.

---

[6] Adaptation theory by Brickman, Coates and Bulman in American Psychology Association.

[7] Dutch Postcode Lottery study by Kuhn, Kooreman Soetevent, Kapteyn.

Magic Mindset for Money

Principle 1: Always Look Ahead
Principle 2: See with Your Mind, Not with Your Eyes
Principle 3: Want It Badly and Believe It Is Coming

Tips

1. Take inspiration from real-life heroes who overcame worse situations than what you are in right now.
2. Shift your mindset from that of worry to that of abundance.
3. Remember that money isn't everything and cannot buy everlasting happiness.

Steps to Worry Less about Money:

1. Take Stock
2. Analyse Expenses and Cut Down

    a) Spend less
    b) Catch little things
    c) Save electricity
    d) Make a monthly budget
    e) Use only cash
    f) Cut your losses

3. Try a Different Thing
4. Think Creatively
5. Create Passive Streams of Income
6. Do More with What Is Already There
7. Let It Go: Believe and Trust

6

Magic Mindset for Relationships

We're the choices we make.
—Francesca in *The Bridges of Madison County*

THE OTHER DAY, CURLED UP ON MY SOFA, I WAS ENGROSSED in a Danish political drama on TV, *Borgen*, about a woman, Birgitte, becoming prime minister. She and her husband have an understanding—that they each take five years by turns to focus on their career while the other one focuses on running the home and taking care of the children. When her husband jokingly asks Birgitte what would happen if he was offered the position of CEO of Microsoft while it was his turn to manage the home, Brigitte laughingly says he would have to turn it down.

In another instance, when Birgitte is getting ready to go on national television for the final debate, she struggles to get into a skirt, even as the taxi pulls up outside. Her eleven-year-old daughter tells her father, 'You have to tell her that she is too fat to fit into the skirt.' Birgitte struggling with the zip, leaves it open and covers it with her jacket. She then asks her husband what he thinks. He asks her if she wants the loving version or the truth.

Brigitte says, 'The truth.'

Her husband says, 'There are about five kilos between you and the black suit.'

Birgitte then asks for the loving version, and her husband says the cleaners shrunk the suit and it is their fault.

Birgitte and her husband tackle big issues with honesty, and yet, there is kindness. They communicate with each other constantly and back it up with gestures of kindness. This is the 'magic mindset' of relationships—where there is honesty, communication and the willingness to understand and see it from the other person's point of view.

Principle 1: Communicate, Communicate and Add Some Kindness

While fictional TV show couples can 'communicate' and 'talk' about issues, real-life couples who can do that are rare. When we come back from work, tired and stressed after a long day, we want to feel welcomed and happy. If the other person too has had a stressful day, both end up ordering out some dinner and watching the television till they are exhausted and go to bed.

Even in bed, there's mostly the interference of mobile phones. We're truly not 'with each other' even when we are physically next to each other. We're tied to our work, tethered by the internet connectivity, 24/7. While we might talk to each other (What is for breakfast? Do you need help with the dishes?), rare is the couple in a long-term relationship that actually communicates.

In our home, we have a simple rule that we all follow: No phones allowed at the dining table. We also have a rule that everyone in the family will eat together if they happen to be home. If one of the family members is caught up in a call, the others wait till they are done. Needless to say, most of our conversations happen around the dining table.

If communication has to improve between people, we need to make a conscious effort. When my children were younger, we would introduce them to 'thinking questions' at the dining table. The questions would be all kinds—playful ones, serious ones that required thought or just ones that aroused curiosity. Sometimes, we would have a 'fun facts' day and each person had to talk about some fun fact they had discovered. Mealtimes are always happy times. We'd followed this rule long before we had children, and after they were born, we simply decided to continue it and modified it a bit to make it more fun for the kids.

As adults, we have mostly forgotten how to have fun! Most of my friends who are married or in long-term relationships tell me that even when they do talk about something, it is usually 'heavy topics', like politics.

The way in which we communicate with each other also plays a great role in relationships. According to several published studies, communication occupies a central role in a relationship. Happy marriages (or long-term relationships) are distinguished from unhappy ones by the ratio of positive to negative behaviour in the relationship. When we are unhappy, we communicate differently than when we are happy and content. Even if we do not say anything, our body language gives us away.

If we are equipped with 'good communication patterns', we tend to feel positive in our relationships. We know deep down that whatever the issue, we can talk it over and sort it out. But if the communication patterns are negative, then we go around in circles, discussing the same things over and over.

In order to communicate well, we need to put ourselves in the other person's shoes and see things from their point of view. It helps to rephrase what we think the other person is saying. A good communication practice is to say, 'What I hear is _____' (fill in with what the other person has said). This gives them confidence that we have heard and understood what they are communicating.

The other thing to remember is to state the issue and not blame the person. If we are annoyed that the other person leaves wet towels on the floor, rather than saying, 'You always do this; I have reminded you many times,' we must try saying, 'When the wet towels are left on the floor, it makes me sad because I like a tidy room.' In the second way of communicating, the person doesn't feel blamed. We have stated the problem and expressed our feelings without hurting them, and thus we have a higher chance of success.

Sometimes, a couple just works out their own ways of communicating with each other, and that is fine too. I've been married for twenty-five years, and my husband and I can read each other's minds! We don't have to say a word to know whether the other person is in a good mood or not. If one of us is in a bad mood, the other one leaves them alone till it has passed. Knowing when to keep quiet is an art and a skill in a marriage.

Principle 2: Take Out the Time to Put In the Work

James Redfield in his book *The Celestine Prophecy* says:

> When love first happens, the individuals are giving each other energy unconsciously and both people feel buoyant and elated. That's the incredible high we call being 'in love.' Unfortunately, once they expect this feeling to come from another person, they cut themselves off from the energy in the universe and begin to rely even more on the energy from each other—only now there doesn't seem to be enough and so they stop giving each other energy and fall back into their dramas in an attempt to control each other and force the other's energy their way.

What Redfield essentially suggests is that when a couple is deeply in love, they begin relying more and more on each other, to fulfil all their needs—emotional, physical and perhaps spiritual too. I know many couples who 'adjust their needs' after they get married, because they badly want the relationship to work.

We're always told that all long-term relationships, especially marriages, are a 'give and take'. But often what happens is that patterns begin to form, where one person gives and gives and the other person keeps 'taking'. Both parties are usually not aware because this happens over a period of many years. Both end up dissatisfied. The *giver* feels depleted, and the *taker* wonders why the giver isn't as enthusiastic or as much fun as they were before.

I like to think of a relationship as a plant; both go through different stages of growth. The plant needs the right amount of sunlight, fertilizer and water to grow. Once a plant has given enough flowers from a stem, we need to 'deadhead' it. We need to weed it regularly. The branches need to be trimmed. Similarly, a relationship too needs different inputs that must be adjusted according to the personality types of the two people involved in it. Relationships need constant care as well as some amount of 'healthy neglect'. It must be natural and yet it needs 'direction'.

The key to a positive and happy relationship lies in understanding the needs of our partner, and our partner reciprocating the same.

Principle 3: Bring Back the Fun

In light of a constantly evolving relationship and the other stressors we face on a day-to-day basis in life, how do we keep up the mindset that our relationships first began with, when everything was wonderful? Are there any specific things we can do to keep our relationships fresh and loving?

The answer to this is not so simple or straightforward. If the relationship has been neglected for many years, it will take a lot of effort from both sides to set it right. If there are serious issues, then we must communicate them with our partner when both people are relaxed.

But if there are no serious issues, and it is just that things don't have the same freshness that they used to have, maybe the relationship needs some *dusting and polishing*.

Exercise 6a

If you are not entirely happy with your relationship and believe that it can be better, then write down the main complaints you have.

Exercise 6b

Write down 5 wonderful things that you appreciate about your partner.

Exercise 6c

Write down the possible ways that you can communicate, with kindness, to your partner the problems you have in your relationship. Remember to start by appreciating them for the nice things that they do.

Tips to Rekindle Fun and Love

1. Understand Your Partner's Needs

In the initial days of love, when everything is new, the flame of love burns very bright. We are still discovering things about our partner; we do not know them fully. But as months or years pass, we get used to their habits and behaviour. We learn certain patterns and we stick to these patterns of behaviour. As time passes, we become very comfortable in our relationship. We presume that we know the other person very well. This is the danger zone where a certain amount of 'taking-the-other-person-for-granted' can creep in. We may neglect to notice things about our partner. We may be so busy in our careers, raising a family, running a home that nurturing this plant called 'relationship' is forgotten.

In Gary Chapman's *Five Love languages,* he says that the way people express love is different. For one person, taking out the garbage every morning might be an expression of love; but for another person, their partner gifting them flowers would count as an expression. Yet another person might need to hear words of affirmation to feel loved, but another might be very uncomfortable in actually uttering those words. Chapman says that we learn to speak our 'primary love language' in childhood based on how our parents expressed love to us, and it is very rarely that both people in a relationship speak the same love language.

Hence, if we want to communicate positively to our partner, we must understand their primary love language and we constantly practise it to nurture our relationships. We need to keep an eye out for instances when our partner's face lights up with love, and we need do those things more often.

2. Make Many Positivity Deposits

In some ways, relationships are like plants, but in other ways they are also like banks. Any kind and loving act we do towards our partner will go into 'deposits'. Each time we have a fight or say something mean to them, it will go into 'withdrawals'. For the relationship to be rich and growing, the balance of accounts should always be positive.

Here it is important to ensure that the 'deposit' we make is viewed as that by the other person as well. Thus, if we get flowers for our partner, we might assume that we are making a 'deposit' but in their eyes, it might not be one. The other person might have preferred us tidying up the apartment instead of getting flowers. We need to pay attention to what love language our partner speaks. We then need to make a deposit in that currency.

If you do not know or are unsure about what makes your partner feel loved, simply ask them! Ask them what their ideal day would be. Then strive to make it happen. Ask them what they would specifically like if you did, and then ensure that you do it.

Exercise 6d

Write down a list, where you do one wonderful thing for your partner every single day of the week. The list could look something like this:

Monday: Take the kids out and give your partner some alone time.

Tuesday: Clean up the apartment before they arrive from work; make it look welcoming.

Wednesday: Offer a back massage.

Thursday: Cook their favourite meal as a surprise.

Friday: Have a long conversation over wine.

Even if a relationship is in not in a great place, making this 'positivity deposit' is increasing the balance of accounts. The other person is bound to notice the change and reciprocate.

The key thing to remember in relationships is this: *You can never withdraw more than you deposit.*

If only one person keeps making the deposits and doesn't get to 'withdraw', that person will eventually stop due to a feeling of depletion and the balance in the accounts will suffer. Therefore, it is important for all parties in a relationship to discuss the idea and be on board. When both people make large amounts of positivity deposits, the relationship grows. A few withdrawals, then, will not harm the relationship.

3. The 'Fun Things' Jar

A few years back, on one of my travels, when I was strolling through the shops in Khan Market in Delhi, I came across a lifestyle store selling quirky objects. One of them was a 'fun things' jar. It was a large glass jar with little cards inside. Inside each card was an activity for the couple to do together. They were colour coded and had various suggestions including naughty ones. One of the things that would go a long way in making a 'positivity' deposit is having a 'fun things' jar. It brings back the playfulness into a relationship. You can plan out activities that both of you enjoy doing together and put it into the jar.

Relationship counsellors say that couples that have many shared interests and hobbies, and engage in them together, have a higher chance of being happy in a long-term relationship than those that do not do anything together.

4. The Kitchen Whiteboard

For a long time now, we have had a whiteboard in our kitchen. The whiteboard can be a great and fun tool for better communication. These days, both my husband and I are working from home in different rooms. We take our breaks at different times, but we leave messages for each other on the board. Our recently graduated children (who are currently living with us) too do the same. Anytime, any of us come to the kitchen, there is always a fun message for someone, in addition to grocery lists. The messages are not always of 'love' and 'happiness'. The other day I requested everyone to clean up after they use the kitchen. My husband expressed how he was annoyed over something, and all of us wrote our apologies.

One can use 'WhatsApp' groups too for the same, but it is a lot more fun with the whiteboard. It is less 'aggressive' and whatever is written can easily be erased. The non-permanence of what is written somehow adds an urgency and uniqueness to it. We also have to write it by hand, rather than type it— and that adds a personal touch. Recently, we also included a 'TFTD' (thought for the day) written by each of us in turn. There are also messages of appreciation and love. It's a fun way to communicate and strengthen bonds.

Keeping a whiteboard in the family will encourage communication. For couples, it can be a novel way to communicate, and who can resist the temptation of scribbling something on a whiteboard? Relationships are constant work. One has to value them enough to communicate constantly, do things differently and inject a little bit of fun by trying new things. Unless we do that, there is a risk of staleness creeping in. The primary foundation of a relationship must be love, trust and respect. If these three things exist in abundance, then the relationship flourishes.

Break-ups and Unrequited Love: The Magic Mindset for Healing

Sometimes, despite all the positivity deposits, and all the efforts that we make, a relationship might just die. The people in the relationship might grow so far apart that the gap cannot be bridged. One person might decide to walk away, leaving the other feeling bewildered and hurt.

Sometimes, two people just grow apart for no obvious reasons. Every single day, the things that we experience change us. We're no longer the person we were at the beginning of the day. Two people react to the same situation in two different ways. To narrate an example from the very poignant 2012 Hindi film *Talash,* the couple loses a child. The husband's way of coping is to turn into a workaholic in the hopes of burying his grief, while the wife consults psychics and mediums hoping to communicate with her child. Both suffer deeply and are devastated, but in different ways. While most couples may not have such a drastic tragedy happen to them, they do undergo losses and face stressors, all of which take their toll.

Everything that happens to us affects us, and as a direct consequence of the changes within us, our relationships too change. The way we connect with others changes too.

As an author who has written several young adult fiction novels, I get mails from thousands of young people seeking my advice. Some of them wonder if they will ever find love. Once I received an angry email from a young lady, about how she felt cheated because she would never find love like the protagonist of my book! In this regard, I would like to emphasize that true love rarely happens when we are actively chasing it. It often creeps up on us, unnoticed. We must be patient. The best thing we can do is lead a meaningful life in the meanwhile.

I am a big believer in the Law of Attraction. What we express gratitude for, multiplies. We need to be grateful for the love we already have in our lives—be it from our parents, or our friends or even a pet. But if we express our love for someone and they reject us, or say that they don't feel the same way about us, it is going to hurt. Rejections and break-ups hurt. In many ways, the pain is something incomparable. We fall into a hopeless state and everything looks bleak. Often it feels physical—like a stone in the heart. All we can think of is the person who isn't in our life any more. We replay in our mind the things we said, the things they said and what could have been done differently. We bristle at the unfairness of the treatment we have received.

The main thought that runs through anyone's mind after a break-up is, 'How in the world could they do this to me? Especially after all I have done for them.'

We drown in the emotional turmoil, unable to understand how things could go so wrong, when once upon a time, we both were so deeply in love. Mostly, relationships fail for reasons beyond our control. They end because they had come with an expiry date. We have a hard time accepting that everything need not last forever, and we are deeply disappointed because we are cheated out of our 'happily-ever-after', especially if we have put in the effort to do 'all the right things'.

There are no easy ways to get over someone. It is going to hurt, and it will hurt for a long time—maybe months, maybe years. But with time, the pain will lessen, or at the very least, it will lose its sharp edges. We grow from failed relationships.

We become better versions of ourselves, ready to love in a different way, the next time someone worthy of our affection comes along. Though it may seem impossible in the moment, when we are hurting so much, things do change.

There are some things that we can do when a relationship has failed and we have decided to part ways. We must remember that healing is a long process, but we can make it slightly more bearable using coping strategies. The following are some tips on using the magic mindset to get over a heartbreak.

1. Unfollow Everywhere

Very often, people spend time stalking their ex and reopening old wounds after a relationship has ended. If we truly desire to heal, the best option is to treat it as a closed door. Looking at their pictures, and worrying about who they are meeting and what they are doing is a drain of our precious energy and will harm us. We must harden our heart and block them!

If we are going through a break-up and have decided to move on, we must make our mind strong. No matter what the temptation, we cannot look back. This is a difficult choice for many, and it requires a good amount of will power. Lean on a trusted friend or a confidant if need be. The mind is energetically connected to the person, and it will take a while to not think about them. But just take one day at a time. Let the goal be, 'I will not look at their profile today.' The next day, make the same resolution again. Before you realize, a week will have passed, then a month, then a year. By then, you will probably be in a much stronger position.

2. Cut the Cord: A Mental Exercise

Many years back, a person I considered very close decided to part ways with me. She gave no satisfactory explanations. I tried my hardest to find out what happened. I wondered about what I had said to hurt her. Many emails and phone calls later, I knew she didn't want to keep in touch with me. Since it was a friendship of many years and we'd been close enough where we even visited each other with our families and stayed in each other's homes, it was very painful for me.

I came across a mental exercise that helped me to heal. Doing the exercise helped me a lot in letting go of the painful feelings of losing my friend. I wished her well each time I meditated. It helped me heal. We're not in touch any more, and it has been many years. I don't feel bad about losing the friendship, and I have moved on with my life.

An Exercise to Help You Heal from a Broken Relationship

1. Go to a room or space where you will not be disturbed for about fifteen minutes.
2. Sit or lie down in a comfortable position and close your eyes.
3. Take thirty deep breaths, relaxing deeper and deeper with each breath. Inhale though the nose to a count of four and exhale through the mouth to a count of six. Keep doing this till you reach a state of deep relaxation.

4. Imagine energy cords going from your physical body and connecting to your friend's physical body. If the relationship is one that has been existing for many years, then the cords are entangled and intertwined tightly together, so much so that you have no idea which cord is whose.
5. Now imagine a giant golden scissor, cutting these cords in the middle. Snap. The cords are cut.
6. Imagine 'grounding' your own cords. Tie them together mentally and bury them deep down in the soil, going deeper and deeper into the earth.
7. Visualize a bright light emanating from the earth, encircling you, filling you with calmness and peaceful energy. You are now ready to let go of the person.
8. Say to the universe:
   'I hereby release all attachments I had with _____.'
   'I wish _____ well and hope they are happy on their chosen path.'
9. Once you complete this exercise, lie or sit in silence for a few minutes. (You might have to repeat this exercise a few times, especially if you are new to visualizing and energy mediations.)

This visualization exercise creates positivity and good vibes, where we acknowledge that something has ended, we're grateful for whatever lessons we learnt from the experience, and we're now ready to travel down a new path.

3. Fill the Void

When we had been spending weekends and all our free time with the person who has now parted ways, it might seem daunting to suddenly have whole weekends empty. But we must look on the bright side. This is the time we can attend a dance workshop or go go-carting, or do something that we always wanted to do but never got to because of our partner.

Someone I know ended their marriage of twenty-eight years. They had been slowly growing apart and staying together 'for the sake of the children'. Once the children grew up, there was nothing holding them together any more. The wife told me that it was like she was rediscovering herself. For the first few months, she was busy as she had to find a home, move by herself and do a lot of things on her own in a long time. She leaned on her friends, cried for weeks and then decided to stop feeling sorry for herself. She is now in a happier place, and her home is gorgeous, filled only with the things that bring her joy. She said she has never felt this light in her life. She has joined a fitness class, she meets friends, she has time to read and cycle—all of which she had put on hold to direct her energy towards 'compromising and adjusting', trying to make their marriage work for so many years. The more she connected with her inner self, the happier she felt. It did take time. But she eventually got to the place where she is now content and peaceful. She says that while it was painful in the beginning, deciding to part ways was the best thing that ever happened to her.

We have for many years been conditioned to think that once we have found 'The One', we should compromise and make it work. Often, this comes at the cost of making ourselves the last priority. We then become beaten down, unhappy versions of ourselves, not fully living our lives or doing what we want to do. Engaging in new activities which we've wanted to try renews a sense of purpose and fills us with enthusiasm for life. It brings back the positivity.

4. Give It Time

A quote I read on the internet said, 'Be 1 per cent better than yesterday'. I found this to be a very motivating quote that can be applied to all aspects of life. What a wonderful thing to strive for! This is a tiny, executable action that can make us feel better with each passing day.

Ending a relationship is like having a fall. How hard we fall and hurt depends on how deep the relationship was. Sometimes, for the other person, it might not have been as deep as it was for us. It hurts even more then. When we sustain a fracture, the doctor puts the affected part in a cast so that it can rest until the bone mends. The rest is mandatory. Even after it heals, we have to go easy on the bone that has just healed. We have to be careful to not lift heavy weights and take extra precautions so we don't end up injuring it again.

It's the same with the heart. If it has been bruised, we need to rest. We need to go easy on ourself and do what feels good—stay back at home, not talk to anyone you do not want to, eat tubs of ice cream, watch movies.

Many people write to me after a broken relationship. They are in so much pain that they don't know what to do. They expect a quick solution. There isn't any. The only thing you can do is give it time. Just like a plant can't be rushed to grow, the new you will take time to emerge. The 'broken' you is now transforming. You cannot see the changes as they are so subtle, and much beneath the surface. But make no mistake—*you are healing*. When you emerge, you will be a stronger, smarter and, hopefully, a kinder version of yourself.

If you are in a relationship, ensure that it is a happy one. If you are in one that needs repairs, reach out to your partner and talk about fixing things. Do not let wounds and regrets fester. If the relationship makes you very unhappy and it is beyond repair, consider ending it. Understand and accept that healing will take years and is a long process. You deserve happiness and positivity in all aspects of your life. You owe it to yourself to lead a life of contentment and joy.

Magic Mindset for Relationships

Principle 1: Communicate, Communicate and Add Some Kindness
Principle 2: Take Out the Time to Put In the Work
Principle 3: Bring Back the Fun

Tips to Rekindle Fun and Love

1. Understand Your Partner's Needs
2. Make Many Positivity Deposits
3. The 'Fun Things' Jar
4. The Kitchen Whiteboard

Tips to Get Over a Break-up

1. Block Everywhere
2. Cut the Cord: A Mental Exercise
3. Fill the Void
4. Give It Time

7

Magic Mindset for Good Health

When health is absent, wisdom cannot reveal itself, art cannot manifest, strength cannot fight, wealth becomes useless, and intelligence cannot be applied.

—Herophilus

RECENTLY, I RAN A POLL ON MY SOCIAL MEDIA TO ASK people whether they wished to lead a healthier lifestyle than they currently did. Almost 88 per cent of the people voted 'yes', as they were unhappy about the life that they were leading. The high figures of unsatisfied people came as a surprise to me. When I asked what was it that they wanted to change about their current lifestyles, I noticed a few things patterns. Some wished to lose weight, some wanted to wake up earlier, some wanted to reduce screen time, some wanted to follow a regular exercise regimen and some just wanted to be 'less lazy'. Most people knew what they wanted to do but felt 'stuck' in their current situation. A 100 per cent of the people voted yes when asked if they believed that taking care of their health was important. Mahatma Gandhi had said that it is health that is real wealth, not pieces of gold and silver, and from the poll I ran, it was evident that everyone agreed.

Individual Health: The Current Scenario in India

According to a 2019 report on the health of the Indian populaition, published by GOQii[8], a California-based healthcare platform, the number of diabetes cases in the under-45 age group has spiked by 40 per cent, and the instances of high blood pressure have gone up by 90 per cent. The overweight population has increased to 57 per cent. One out of every four Indians reports aches and pains of some kind. One out of four also suffers from acute stress. The pandemic has only made the situation worse. According to multiple reports in various newspapers, one out of every four Indians requires medical intervention to manage their stress and mental health.[9]

While we all know *how* to take care of our health, what we are lacking is the motivation to do it. We're stuck in our

---

8   Source: https://goqii.com/blog/lifestyle-diseases-an-epidemic-among-young-indians/
    Source: https://goqii.com/blog/tag/fitness-and-lifestyle-in-india/
    Source: https://www.livemint.com/insurance/news/health-insurance-a-must-to-combat-the-rise-in-lifestyle-diseases-1567068428855.html

9   Source: https://economictimes.indiatimes.com/magazines/panache/mental-health-in-india-7-5-of-country-affected-less-than-4000-experts-available/articleshow/71500130.cms

routine, wanting to make a change but somehow unable to. We procrastinate, saying that we will exercise 'tomorrow', but before we realize many 'tomorrows' have passed, and many months, maybe years have gone by. We set the intention the previous night that we will wake up early, but when the alarm on the phone goes off, we hit that snooze button, intending to sleep for just ten more minutes; but when we open our eyes, an hour has passed. We want to eat healthier, but when we have our tea, it is hard to resist that samosa or pack of potato chips to go with it, especially when everyone else seems to be enjoying it. 'Just this one time won't make a difference,' we tell ourselves, and repeat the same behaviour every day.

My Own Story: A Perspective

I was raised in a house where taking care of one's health was of paramount importance. My parents were extremely conscious of how a faulty diet led to lifestyle diseases—something that could easily be avoided by choosing the right things to eat. Both of them were on the same page when it came to diet. They would eat simple, fresh food made with locally available ingredients. Having grown up in homes that did not have refrigerators, they believed in cooking just the right quantity needed for a meal. They detested refrigerating and reheating leftovers. Cooking in small amounts, they always ate delicious, piping hot, fresh meals with locally available ingredients. Since my parents loved gardening, much of the time, these ingredients were homegrown and organic. Long before 'organic' and 'buy local' became fashionable, my parents were following it.

My father used to say, 'Eat to live, do not live to eat.' He and my mother were great believers in the concept of 'fresh air and exercise cures almost everything' and these were phrases I heard constantly. They went for long walks daily. My grandparents too believed in the same. Neither of my grandparents ever visited a hospital all their lives! My parents, too, have very rarely been to doctors, except for their annual check-ups.

Observing them, I automatically understood that the main thing for good health is a good diet. If we eat right, it takes care of most lifestyle diseases. Having been raised in such an environment, I presumed this was the norm and this was how it was for everyone. Naively, I believed that everyone led similar lives. I didn't think much about the life my parents led nor did I see it as 'extraordinary'.

When I was about fourteen, I was invited for a meal at a friend's place. The food served was rich and the items were far too many. In comparison, what we ate normally at home was frugal. My friend said this was their everyday fare. I was also surprised to discover that they cooked all their food in ghee—something that was never done at my place. The way we lived was almost spartan compared to theirs.

My friend's father had lifestyle diseases ranging from hypertension to diabetes. Her mother suffered from arthritis. My friend explained that it was 'culturally an impossible thing' to eat food that was less rich. She said that in their families, the notion was that it is only the old people who 'couldn't eat food cooked in ghee' and had to forgo this pleasure. Her parents would say, 'We can enjoy life now; we aren't old yet.' Just like my parents believed in eating healthy and exercising, her parents believed in 'enjoying life' by eating whatever satisfied the palate.

Inadvertently, my parents had cultivated in me the *magic mindset of health*—to eat right, and to exercise. It is ingrained in me, and I cannot imagine a life without exercise.

Even if we haven't been raised with this mindset, it can be cultivated.

When it comes to the magic mindset for health, there is really no 'magic'. There are just two principles one must always remember:

Principle 1: Eat right
Principle 2: Exercise

Exercise 7a

Do you wish to be healthier? If so write down all the reasons why you would like to be healthier. Example: Felt more energetic, Free of body pains, fitter body etc.

Exercise 7b

Write down why you are unable to achieve the above goals. Where do you falter?

Cultivating a Magic Mindset for Health

There's only one way to lead a healthier lifestyle: we must make up our mind and firmly stick to it. If we wish to be healthier, we have to make it a priority. We have to devote time to it. It needn't be a sudden or a drastic change. But little things done every single day go a long way in making a positive change towards your health.

There are a few things we can do to improve our lifestyle, leading to better health and a positive mindset.

1. Waking Up Earlier

One of the key benefits of waking up an hour earlier than we usually do is that it adds time at our disposal—time that we could use in productive ways, perhaps to do an exercise regimen or to do yoga, or simply to go for a walk around the neighbourhood. While in theory, it sounds great, implementing it is hard.

Like most people, I detest waking up early. I live in Bengaluru, where the weather is pleasant throughout the year because of the high elevation. This weather is sometimes called a 'holiday climate' as the natural inclination is to curl up under a duvet and sleep for a bit longer. During winters, I sleep till around 7.30 a.m. But during summer, I am up at 6.00 a.m. I was never much of a morning person, but I quickly realized the benefits and I disciplined myself. If you are struggling to wake up in the morning, try the following.

a) **Ask why and write it down:** Set aside some time for deep thinking. Go for a walk, leaving your phone at home, and think about all the reasons why you want to wake up earlier than usual. If you can come up with only a 'generic' reason such as 'all successful people wake up early' or 'because my parents nag me if I sleep late', then you are not going to be motivated to want to do it. Think about what it can do for you. What would you do with that extra time that you would get if you wake up early? How much earlier than usual do you want to wake up? Why? When you are back from your walk, write the answers down on a piece of paper, and stick it where it is visible—perhaps on your wardrobe or above your desk. Make your list as detailed as possible.

When we have a strong, compelling reason and can see the tangible benefits a change will bring, we are more likely to stick to the plan. If we do not write these down, then we only have a vague idea in our head. But when we do list them, the benefits are visible and will goad us to take action. If we live with other people, they can see our intent too and perhaps nudge us towards our goals. Not wanting to 'lose face' in front of them after having declared our intentions can also help us stick to the resolution.

b) **Ease into it slowly**: If you are used to waking up at 8.30 a.m., to set a target of waking up at 6 a.m. is to set yourself up for failure. It is too difficult a task for most people to make such a drastic change. If you set a goal like this, you are unlikely to sustain it for a longer time, unless you have an iron will. What I recommend is easing into your goal slowly. For every alternate day of the week, set the alarm for fifteen minutes earlier. Thus, Tuesdays, Thursdays and Saturdays can be the days that you wake up fifteen minutes earlier than your regular time. On the other four days, you are allowed to wake up at your regular time. Doing this takes off the burden of biting off more than you can chew. By breaking the goal into 'easily doable' segments, you are paving the way for long-term change. After doing this for a week, increase the duration to four days a week. After you achieve that for a week, make it five. Then you can graduate to six days a week. Take Sundays (or any other day) as an off day, when you can sleep for as long as you please. Once you can wake up fifteen minutes earlier than usual, begin the process all over again! Repeat till you get to the desired time you want to wake up. You could, of course, adjust the time frame as you wish.

When making such changes, the idea is to not make it so hard that we give up in a few days. If we ease into it over a longer period, we can build long-term, permanent changes. These are very small steps that make it easier for us to be consistent with our goals.

c) **Stopping screen time at 8 p.m.:** Several studies have linked the widespread use of electronic devices to poor sleep patterns.[10] Electronic devices emit an artificial blue light, which suppresses the release of melatonin, the sleep-inducing hormone in our bodies. The light emitted from the screen makes us alert and active, and messes with our circadian rhythms. We've all become so connected to our phones, that 'switching off the phone' sounds like an extreme step.

---

10 Source: https://www.sciencedaily.com/releases/2018/11/181127111044.htm
Source: https://www.medicalnewstoday.com/articles/323846

But if you are serious about making a change in your lifestyle, why not give this a try?

Most people say that they are afraid to switch off their phones, because they are scared that they will not be contactable in case of an emergency. But the fact is, many of us are addicted to our phones. If you pause to think about it, in the event of an emergency (the probability of which happening is very minuscule) the person contacting you would probably be able to reach someone close to you, who could then ring your doorbell. Nancy Colier, a psychotherapist and author of several books says that she got a wake-up call when people started asking her for tips to get over their technology addiction. That was when she realized that she was addicted too. Nancy, in order to get over her addiction to the phone, meditated every day and during that brief period, she was able to ward off her phone. But when she finished meditating, the phone got hold of her again and she was at its mercy. I can relate to Nancy's experience, as can so many others. I too tend to be glued to the phone, unless I make a conscious attempt to leave it in another room and stay off it.

If you want less screen time (resulting in better sleep) then there's only one way to do it—going cold turkey. If you are unable to stay away from your phone, hand it over to a family member or a friend and tell them to give it back to you only the next day. You are likely to feel very uncomfortable for a few days. Replace the phone scrolling time with reading. Soon your body's balance will return, and it will start producing melatonin, helping you sleep earlier and resetting your sleep patterns. Added bonus? You will end up reading more!

d) **Get an alarm clock and place it far from the bed:** This is an old trick, but it is a tried-and-tested one. Use an old-fashioned alarm clock rather than your phone. Keep the alarm clock away from your bed—maybe on a table or a desk. You should have to get off the bed to switch it off, forcing you out of the bed. Do not go back to sleep after you have got out of bed. Using an alarm clock also has an added benefit. You are less likely to check your phone as soon as you wake up, since you aren't using it as an alarm clock. Instead, take a few moments to visualize how you want your day to go. If you have meetings, imagine these meetings, in detail, going well. If you have planned to meet friends, imagine the joy and laughter. In your mind, offer a thanks to the universe for gifting you these things. Then have a glass of water and begin your day. This goes a long way in setting a positive tone for the day that lies ahead.

2. Exercising More

Many years back, I visited a beautiful farm with a lot of horses, dogs, poultry and cows. The lady who owned it was energetic, bubbly, jovial and friendly. She also often went riding. When I learnt that she was in her late fifties and a mother to an adult son, I was awestruck. She looked and behaved like she was in her late twenties. I struck up a conversation with her and asked her what she did for her fitness. She said she did not follow any particular regimen. She ate healthy and did a bit of yoga. Being on the farm, she did a lot of physical labour, which she said kept unnecessary thoughts at bay; there was always something that needed her urgent attention on the farm. Impressed by her lifestyle, I resolved that in my fifties that was how I would be. While exercise has always been a part of my life, meeting people like her is motivating and firms up my resolve.

Very often, I share screenshots of the kilometres I cycled or the steps I walked on my social media. I am a person who gets bored easily and if I have to stick to a routine, I have to find ways to make it interesting and fun for me. Every couple of years, I have a new go-to for my fitness. From walking to jogging to Ashtanga Yoga to weight training, I have tried it all over the years and committed to whatever I have chosen. My stint lasted a few months with some forms of exercise, and several years with others. But I have been able to sustain and incorporate at least twenty minutes of exercise every single day into my daily schedule.

Many people write to me asking me how I manage to keep myself motivated to exercise daily. They tell me they want to start exercising but lack motivation. Some of them join a gym in earnest but give up after a few weeks because it is hard.

There are several reasons why many people find it hard to stick to a workout routine. A first step is finding out the root cause. For example, do you have to drive to get to the place of exercise and does traffic irritate you? Do you have a stressful job where you work fifteen hours a day, and after you are done, you just want to relax in front of the television? Did you start an exercise routine but were so sore after a few days that you gave up? Or were you perhaps disappointed when you didn't get to the desired weight level even after you stuck to the exercise and felt discouraged?

Here are a few things to keep in mind if you have trouble exercising regularly.

a) **Each person is different:** A friend of mine, who is a marathon runner, urged me to try running. We used to play basketball together while at school. I was also into competitive athletics back then. He was sure that I would enjoy it. He gave me tips on how to start. He said it was the greatest thing that happened to him, and he spoke about how it changed his life. He said I would start enjoying it, once I started regularly running. Of course, I gave it a try. But after a week, I knew I hated it. I stopped. Running just isn't for me.

You might have started an exercise because your friend recommended it, and it worked for them. While their intentions might be great, what works for them may not work for you. If you dislike it, just stop! Don't feel guilty about it. Accept that each person is different and do not beat yourself up about it. Instead, try a different thing.

b) **Choose something enjoyable:** Don't hesitate to try various things. For a while, I used to follow a YouTube Channel that offered many fitness routines. After a few months, I got bored of it and stopped. When I decided that I wanted to get some kind of exercise on a regular basis, I tried different dance classes in my neighbourhood. I disliked all of them. They were either too much into choreography or would insist on technical details. I wasn't looking to become a dancer! I wanted to find something fun and enjoyable. I then discovered a Zumba class that was exactly what I wanted. It was a small batch of just six to ten people. The instructor was great, and I enjoyed myself. I made new friends, we laughed a lot and all of us looked forward to the next class.

It is only when you try different things that you know what works for you. Sometimes you may know straight away that it isn't for you, after a single class. Sometimes you may discover that you dislike it, after a few weeks. When it ceases to be enjoyable, just stop!

c) **Make it easy to do**: Whatever form of fitness you choose, make it easy for you to *do* it daily. When the goals are too hard, it is more likely that we give up. For example, if we suddenly begin training or exercising for an hour, it might eat into our other activities. Setting easier goals helps us stay motivated. For a few years, I did Ashtanga Yoga every day. The whole routine takes an hour. But there were days when I wasn't motivated at all and couldn't bring myself to do the entire routine. Every person who does Ashtanga starts with a set of two series—Primary A and Primary B. It takes about fifteen minutes to complete both. On the days that I was not motivated, I decided I would do only these two series and end my practice. By making it easier for me, I was able to sustain doing it, even on the days I didn't feel like it. I did not count those days as 'failure'.

So, if you wake up late and can't make it for your forty-five-minute walk, do a fifteen-minute walk instead and count that as 'success'. More 'success' days will help you stay on course, instead of giving up.

d) **Record and share**: I have a yearly planner pinned on the wall next to my desk. It is an ordinary year planner, with small columns for all the months and days of the year. Each day that I exercise, I write it in the planner. I write whatever workout I did that day—walking or cycling or weight training. When I see all the columns filled up, it is extremely motivating for me. When we physically *see* what we have achieved, we are spurred on to stick to it. For me, the small act of writing in that little column on the planner each day is the equivalent of collecting a medal on the victory stand.

I highly recommend a yearly wall planner. Stick it somewhere where you see it daily, and record daily achievements. You could also share what you did with a friend who is encouraging or become exercise buddies. But it is very important to choose a person who has a similar mindset.

e) **Follow people you admire:** I follow a fitness trainer on social media who is in her fifties. She weight trains and posts her daily exercise videos, and I can connect with what she says. I find that when I see other people exercising, I too feel like being active. Being associated with people who are into fitness helps us, encourages us and motivates us.

Choose a fitness account that you feel a personal connection to. The fitness account you choose to follow should make you feel good. There are many accounts that only 'show off' their perfect physiques, achieved through years of sacrifice and hard work, and who knows, maybe steroids too. It might be their main profession—they might be a fitness influencer and they probably make a living out of it. But if it does not add anything of value to your life, don't follow them. Choose a fitness account that resonates with you and motivates you. Don't choose ones that make you feel ashamed of yourself, and especially never choose the ones that 'talk down' to you!

3. Eating Healthier Meals

A friend of mine was desperate to lose weight. She and her husband hired a nutritionist, who drew up an elaborate diet chart for them. Every little morsel that went into her mouth was a planned meal—with time and quantity of food that they should eat. For three weeks, she was really happy. Her meals were on track, she was eating as per the nutritionist's recommendation and had lost two and a half kilos. In the fourth week, she couldn't take it any more. While she was losing weight, she was irritated and grumpy, constantly tired and hungry. She gave up the diet, and almost immediately, put back all the weight she had lost.

Recently, there was a news article about an actress who passed away at a young age and the reports said it was because of a Keto diet. A few years back, there was the fad of 'General Motors' diet, which a friend of mine swore by. These days a lot of people are trying intermittent fasting. Well-meaning friends and new converts extol the virtues of the diet that they have just tried and benefitted from. They strongly recommend it to us. When it comes from a trusted source, we completely believe it and want to try it. But the thing is, what works for one person may not at all work for another.

Moreover, we all crave our 'comfort foods'. For me, it is a simple curd rice and pickle or idli with 'mollaga podi' (also nicknamed gunpowder). For someone else, it might be rajma-chawal or a packet of potato chips. Most diets are so severe in their nature, that they go against what our bodies are used to and crave for. It is difficult to sustain a strict diet for a long period. We need to eat what our bodies are used to, while also making those things healthier and more nutritious.

Here are some practical ways that have helped me a lot. I developed these over many years, after many mistakes. (If you suffer from any health conditions, please do consult your doctor or dietician before you make any changes to your diet.)

a) **Doing a 'meal prep'**: I first came across this term when my son began bodybuilding. Many bodybuilders do it as they eat five to six meals a day. All the meals that are needed for the day are prepared in advance and refrigerated. Since I love fresh food, and I don't want to spend hours in the kitchen, I modified the 'meal prep'. Please note—my diet is predominantly south Indian vegetarian, but you could substitute it with ingredients suited for the cuisine you are used to.

On the weekend, I stock my fridge with the following:

- Freshly ground homemade batter for idlis/dosa.
- Cooked lentils (tur dal, moong dal, etc.)
- Cooked chickpeas.
- Finely chopped onion (I do this every second day)
- Kneaded dough (for chapatis/parathas)
- Boiled potatoes

By keeping the above handy, I am able to whip up a nutritious meal in less than twenty minutes, for a family of four. I also boil half a dozen eggs each morning. Taking adequate protein is extremely important, and most Indian diets do lack protein. I ensure that whenever I eat a meal, 25 per cent of it is food rich in proteins and 25 per cent is food rich in fibre.

There are easy-to-use protein calculators available online, which tell us how much protein our body needs. Using these, you can modify the proportion of protein, fibre and carbs in your diet. If you spend some time studying and understanding how these works, you will be more inclined to keep up your diet. If you keep these few things in mind each time you eat a meal, you will be eating healthy and feeling full.

b) **Clearing out junk food:** When I wanted to lose weight, I cleared out all the junk food (such as 'farsan', 'mixture', sugary biscuits) that used to be in my kitchen. For me, there was unfortunately no way around this. I knew that if I saw that tin of potato chips, I wouldn't be able to resist, so I decided not to keep any at home at all. The first few days were hard; I was used to having some kind of fried snack or chips with my tea. But I stuck to my resolve. If I felt the craving for a snack, I would make myself a tasty 'bhel' consisting of puffed rice, finely chopped onions, coriander, tomato and green chillies. I'd add a dash of chaat masala and some lemon juice. Soon, my body got used to it, and now I no longer crave either the bhel or the snacks. It is amazing how quickly our bodies get used to a new routine, once we stick to it for about ten days.

c) **Fighting cravings with liquids:** Many people are afraid that they will be hungry if they give up the unhealthy snacks that their bodies are used to. My best suggestion for this would be to 'ride the wave'. When I first gave up sugar and all the junk food, my body craved for it. Whenever the craving hit, I decided to have apples and some herbal tea made of tulsi, ginger and turmeric. This ensured that I had 'something to munch on' and also 'something warm to sip on'. Fruits such as apples, bananas and papayas can fill us up. My other 'go-to' to fight the cravings was watermelon juice. I also stocked my fridge with unsweetened soya milk and other unsweetened things that I never in a million years thought I would enjoy.

Tell yourself that you will do it for just three days. Then, when you achieve that, extend it by two more days and keep going. Before you know it, you would have finished ten days. The more you resist the temptation to go back to your old ways, the easier it becomes. If you fail, don't worry. Just start over.

d) **Easy recipes**: Start a recipe book of 'easy and quick' recipes. There are lots of recipes available online. Try ones that appeal to you, look easy and are quick to make. After you try it, make it a point to write it down in your recipe book. You can even do this online and save pictures of the dish you made.

When we record these things, we have a ready reference for next time. I started doing this after I realized that when I tried a recipe found on the internet and then tried to find it a few weeks later to make it again, I had forgotten which one I had followed. Sometimes, the site that I bookmarked for a particular recipe would be gone! After this happened a few times, I began writing down the recipe rather than relying on it being available online.

e) **Reward yourself**: Every three days or so, reward yourself for achieving the task that you have completed—be it waking up early or eating healthy. The key here is not to reward yourself with 'food'. Think of other things that you might have been wanting to do for a while. Now set aside time for that and 'gift' yourself the activity you have been wanting to do.

I take part in art challenges such as Inktober. The theme for each day is given, and artists all over the world draw a picture related to the theme and post it with hashtags. It is something I enjoy immensely. I tell myself that I can do it only if I have worked on my book (or exercised or whatever goal I have set myself for the day). Thus, my art time is my 'reward'. I also give myself small rewards like a set of art pens that I have been wanting to buy.

Reward yourself with things that make you happy. Perhaps it is phone time with a friend. It could be a simple thing—buying a new shade of lipstick or a deodorant. It could even be watching the next episode of your TV show. Whatever it is, allow yourself to 'earn' that reward. This will help you stay motivated.

Magic Mindset During Illness

Despite our best efforts in taking care of our health, we do fall ill. It is a terrible thing to be ill. No matter how positive we are otherwise, when we fall ill, everything is bleak. When we are physically suffering, it is hard to focus on anything else.

We need not deny what we feel. No one has to be positive all the time! When we are ill, we are 'allowed' to feel like we are dying, even if it is just a minor indigestion that will go away soon. It sucks to be unwell—and there's nothing we can do about it.

But wait. While we may not always be able to avoid diseases, there are some things that we can do to feel better.

1. Do Not Search for Symptoms Online

On the desk of my family doctor is a mug that says, 'Please do not confuse your Google Search for my medical degree.' I found it amusing. He told me it was gifted by one of his patients. She came to him because she was convinced that she had cancer. Though he assured her that she did not, she wasn't convinced. Thousands of rupees in a large hospital and many expensive scans later, she came back to my doctor and gifted him the mug. She was perfectly okay; my doctor was right. She swore never to look up symptoms online.

Many of the sites online list a large variety of symptoms. If we read up these symptoms, we are certain to feel scared, because often, the symptoms of a simple ailment and that of a dreaded cancer might be similar. For example, the symptoms of stomach gas can be very similar to that of heart attack. I know someone who was rushed to the hospital because he was convinced he was having a heart attack. After he arrived at the hospital, it turned out that all he needed was an antacid. (Oh, the relief!)

I am not advocating for us to downplay our symptoms. But it is best not to look them up online and draw our own conclusions.

2. See a Reliable Doctor

It is imperative to find a doctor whom we trust. In India, I find that the doctors in large hospitals often prescribe scans and other processes to 'rule out' all possibilities. Chances are, if we go to a large hospital, we will end up paying a hefty bill for a simple ailment.

Try and identify an independent general practitioner whose opinion you can trust. Then consult them for whatever ailments you get. Trust is the most important thing here. The doctor should genuinely care for your well-being and health.

3. Rest and Hydrate

As a rule, whenever I fall ill, I wait for two days before seeing a doctor. In that time, I try home remedies. I almost always recover by the third day. I rarely fall ill, but if I do, I do not get out of bed at all. I rest until I feel that I have recovered. I also ensure that I drink a lot of fluids. If at all I eat, I make sure it is a light diet, easy on my stomach.

My grandmother raised five children. My mother tells me that she used to have a concoction called 'Kashayam', which she brewed out of herbs and spices she grew herself. Any time her children fell ill, her remedy was simple: she would give them a large glass of 'Kashayam' and order them to cover themselves with a blanket right up to the head, and sleep. Magically, they would recover!

The cells in our bodies do have an inherent ability to repair themselves. We need to give them the rest and opportunity to do so when we are ill.

The home remedies are recommended only for minor illnesses. If you think you have a very severe infection, please do see a doctor without delay.

4. Connect with People

A few years ago, I had a health scare. It was an agonizing week as I waited for the biopsy results, which eventually came back negative. I remember waking up with a feeling of dread for a whole week. I spoke to my best friend, and she too was terrified for me. She made all kinds of promises to God and prayed for my recovery.

I could cope with the stress and the anxiety as I had various people to talk to. Another friend of mine went through a similar health scare. She was convinced she had cancer, and she suffered from anxiety and panic attacks till the diagnosis came. I would speak to her every day and tell her it was nothing. When the results came, it turned out to be something minor, which was easily fixed with medication.

When we fall ill and have to get tests done, the time we spend agonizing over what it could possibly be is excruciating. It helps to have people to talk it over with. When we are ill, we must reach out and speak to people and not hesitate to say that we need help. But we must be careful to stay away from people who make us feel worse!

Our health is one of our greatest assets. The irony is that most of us take our bodies for granted. It is only when we are ill that we realize the value of good health. We've all experienced moments during illnesses when we feel like we are dying. After we've recovered, we feel silly to have felt that way. But in the moment, the excruciating agony of helplessness takes over our minds.

When it comes to health, we have two choices.

1. We can adopt a healthy habit, eat sensibly and avoid all the lifestyle diseases to the maximum extent possible.
2. We can ignore our health and trust that it will take care of itself.

Either way, we will live! Life will go on. But the kind of life we live depends entirely on us and what we desire.

Remember, we are what we do! Tomorrow, we will be whatever we did today. Our tomorrow can become better as a result of all the actions we take today.

Note: The above has been written from the perspective of people who aren't afflicted with serious illnesses like cancer. In case you have a chronic health condition, I recommend the following motivational books from people who have fought these diseases and survived:

Close to the Bone, Lisa Ray
The Test of My Life, Yuvraj Singh
Healed, Manisha Koirala
Uplift, Barbara Delinsky

Magic Mindset for Health

Principle 1: Eat right
Principle 2: Exercise

Tips

1. Waking Up Earlier

a) Ask why and write it down
b) Ease into it slowly
c) Stopping screen time at 8 p.m.
d) Get an alarm clock and place it far from the bed

2. Exercising More

a) Each person is different
b) Choose something enjoyable
c) Make it easy to do
d) Record and share
e) Follow people you admire

3. Eating Healthier Meals

a) Doing advance meal prep
b) Clearing out junk food
c) Fighting cravings with liquids
d) Easy recipes
e) Reward yourself

Magic Mindset During Illness

1. Do Not Search for Symptoms Online
2. See a Reliable Doctor
3. Rest and Hydrate
4. Connect with People

PART 3

Sustaining the Magic Mindset: Fight the Drains

8

Magic Mindset and Awareness

Without water drops, there can be no oceans; without steps, there can be no stairs; without little things, there can be no big things!

—Mehmet Murat Ildan

WE MAY BE HAPPY WITH OUR FINANCES; OUR relationships might be great; and our health may be perfect. Yet, for most of us, even when the larger aspects of life are well and in place, there are things that make us feel drained. They might not be what we view as 'major problems', but the toll they take on us every day eventually wears us down.

Often, these are things that we don't even imagine are a strain on us. Many years back, I had a friend who would call me up daily, just to talk. The phone calls lasted for almost an hour. She was tired of her marriage, and she had many fights with her husband. Every day, she had a new problem or situation to discuss. No matter what 'solution' or advice I came up with, she would find some excuse about why that wouldn't work. After several such sessions, I realized she only wanted to dump her problems on me. She wasn't going to leave her husband or take any action. She didn't really want solutions. She just wanted someone to rant to. While I was being a good friend, it was taking a toll on me. It drained me and left me feeling uneasy. Never once did this person ask me if I was free, or if she was taking up my time. She just presumed it was okay. It took me a few months to get rid of that friendship. I felt light and happy when it ended. I had no idea how taxing it had been to constantly listen to her until I stopped.

The Cost of Interactions

Every interaction that we have with others—whether it is in person, or whether on social media—has an impact on us. We might spend about forty-five minutes to an hour on social media, or as little as ten minutes. Regardless, every little bit of content that we engage with, influences our emotions. We might get enraged by a tasteless comment someone has made about an issue we care about deeply. A picture of something cruel and sad that happened in some corner of the world may disturb us greatly. We assume that once we exit social media and get on with our daily lives, these issues are out of our system. But the things we read and the people we engage with leave a lasting impact and slowly drains our energy, even when we don't realize it because we are not consciously making choices.

When I asked my readers what are the things that make it hard for them to be positive, I received a variety of answers ranging from exam and interview stress to old memories playing on a loop to situations over which they have absolutely no control. No matter what the 'little drains' are, there are ways to fix them by taking certain steps and modifying how we behave in those situations. Over the next few chapters, I will share some tips on cultivating a 'magic mindset' for such situations.

9

The Magic Mindset for Situations Beyond Our Control

> When something bad happens, you have three choices—let it define you, destroy you or strengthen you.
>
> —*Zombieland*

THERE ARE SOME SITUATIONS WE SIMPLY HAVE NO control over, where we find ourselves in a helpless position. Let me share a few real-life situations faced by people who reached out to me.[11]

Tanushree lost her job just before the pandemic started. The company she was working for was taken over by another firm, and her role was made redundant. Single, in her late

---

11 The names and other identifying details have been changed.

thirties, Tanushree had been planning to take a loan and buy a flat before she was let go. She was forced to shelve her plans and move back to her parent's place in a hill town because she couldn't find another job. She wrote to me about how she feels stuck, and though she has sent out many applications, no suitable opportunities have come her way.

Dhanya is doing her post-graduation and wants to be economically independent. While her parents are pressurizing her to get married, she is afraid to tell them that she is in love with someone else. She feels stressed as her parents keep nagging her to get married and 'settle down'. They tell her that her classes are 'only online', and she can continue after she gets married.

Vivek comes from a middle-class family. He is in his late twenties. Through his well-paying job, he had saved up enough to pay for a college in Australia for higher education. But soon after he paid the fees and quit his job, the pandemic hit. The course was stalled and his company refused to take him back.

Selvam has recently graduated from a reputed engineering college but is unable to find a suitable job. He has been rejected by four firms he has interviewed with.

We all know people who are in situations like the ones Tanushree, Dhanya, Vivek and Selvam are in. The pandemic has brought drastic changes to our lives. A friend tells me that she went to a mall in her neighbourhood after five months. It was a surreal experience as there was no one there. She has been going to the same mall for a decade. Before, at any point of time, day or night, there were always thousands of people there. But this time, she could spot only six people. By the time she left, there was nobody.

I feel the same way when I drive out on Bengaluru roads these days. Before, traffic congestion was the norm; now the roads are all deserted. Within a three-kilometre radius from my home, I have spotted at least fifteen 'To Let' signs. With work from home becoming the norm, many people have left the city and returned to their hometowns.

New Realities

Many of my friends who are in corporate jobs tell me that their companies are cutting the space they rent by a third. Having discovered through social media that productivity is not affected even if people work from home, many companies are choosing to save on rent by surrendering the space. The pandemic has changed our outlook, our lifestyle and our world views. No one knows what the future is going to look like.

The depressing situation of job losses and unemployment is exacerbated by the incessant news of suicides and deaths. I recently received a message from a management committee of my neighbouring residential complex group, where we were told about a COVID case in the neighbourhood. The message detailed how the household was quarantined, and outlined the precautions we must all take. Then, a few days later, a person from that house passed away. Even though I did not know them at all, I was overwhelmed by sadness. Each time I pass that house, I feel sad for the people inside, though I have never met them and don't even know their names. Almost everyone I speak to has a similar story to share. They know someone who has lost a loved one to the pandemic or have themselves witnessed death.

Before the pandemic hit us, when we heard the news of a disaster, we felt sad but it did not overwhelm us; we could distance ourselves. But these days it seems like the burden is too much to bear. I have had friends reach out to me because they lost their mother but couldn't even be there for the last rites because of restrictions. The general mood is that of pessimism as death and economic devastation consumes the world. Our emotional straws are stretched gossamer thin. Even a tiny failure becomes a boulder crushing us, because of the hopelessness we are surrounded with. How is it even possible to 'be positive' when we have totally no control over the situation?

We would all love to be positive and pretend that everything is fine, but not acknowledging the stress and trying to suppress it will only lead to mental health issues in the long run.

Principle 1: Accept the Feelings

Some people like to point out that others have it worse. They tell us that we must be grateful because we have food to eat, a roof over our heads and love in our lives. But other people's misery does not negate what *we* feel.

It is perfectly okay to feel sad about one's life or plans that didn't work out. We are allowed to feel what we feel. One of the most important steps in making a change towards positivity is accepting what we feel instead of suppressing it. We need to allow ourselves to experience sadness and be with it for a while. What we feel is valid and real to us. It is not always possible to 'look at the bright side' and be grateful for the things we have.

Once we have accepted the sadness, lived with it for a while, processed it and allowed it to be, then we prepare for the next steps to make a change for the better. Just like Tanushree, Dhanya, Vivek and Selvam, many of us are in situations that are perhaps out of our control. However, we can take certain steps to change our mindset.

Exercise 8a

Write down a situation that frustrates you, that you have absolutely no control over. Write down why you have no control over it.

Principle 2: Take Baby Steps

When we have no control over the situation, all we can do is take baby steps and go through it one day at a time. We have to do what is expected of us in the day and refuse to think about what is in store. Worrying about what we cannot change will only frustrate us further.

When I lost my father and was plunged into extreme grief, there was nothing I could do to immediately feel better. But as days turned into months and months turned into years, I learnt to cope. Looking back, I now know that I was taking baby steps towards healing and acceptance. When we cannot change a situation, there are small things that we can do to cope better.

I call it the practice of ACDC: Acknowledge, Change, Detach and Create. We do not necessarily have to go through *all* the steps. How one does it will depend on their level of sadness and their state of mind. The key is to adapt the practice to suit our needs. Feel free to modify, adapt and change any step in a manner that works for *you*, but remember, merely reading it and doing nothing will not help.

1. Acknowledge

Often in life, we try to resist the feeling of grief or anger or hurt. We don't allow ourselves to feel it fully because it is an uncomfortable feeling. We look for instant ways to distract ourselves by watching a movie, calling a friend, reaching for a drink or anything else that makes us feel better.

Don't. We must allow ourselves to sit with these feelings and express them.

Psychologists stress the importance of acknowledging emotions. No one likes feeling sad or helpless, so the easiest thing is to try and push it away. This is also true when it comes to confronting somebody. Most people hate confrontations. When I was younger, I would do anything to avoid confrontations as they made me anxious. I ended up tolerating a lot because of it. But over time, the situation I refused to address only grew. The problem never went away. Now that I am older, I no longer go to extreme lengths to avoid confrontations. I have learnt to handle it. We must learn to deal with the uncomfortable emotions we experience—grief, anger, helplessness.

Pushing away emotions is no better than drowning our feelings in alcohol. It is a temporary fix; the alcohol takes care of pain for a moment, but in the long run, we end up needing more and more of it to feel better and the problem still remains.

If you want to acknowledge difficult emotions, try talking out loud to yourself or writing things down.

Exercise 8b

Describe how the situation you mentioned in exercise 8a makes you feel. Express everything that you feel.

Your answers above could also be verbally stated. Something like, 'I am feeling sad because I feel alone and no one understands me', or 'I am feeling angry because this person behaved in a manner that I never expected them to.'

It is important to *express* what we feel. By letting it outside, we define what we experience. For instance, if you have a close friend, you could tell them what you are going through and ask them to just listen. If you do not want to share your grief, you can write down your feelings for your eyes only.

When we have trouble expressing our feelings, the following exercise can help. (You may skip it if you've already done exercise 8b.)

Exercise 8c

1. What am I feeling? Am I angry? Am I hurt? Do I feel slighted? Do I feel ignored? Do I feel helpless?
2. Write down the cause of what created that feeling.

I am _____ because _____ happened.

Or

I am _____ because _____ behaved in a way that hurt me.

Once you have expressed it, you have 'released' it.

Identifying what we feel, acknowledging it and expressing it out loud are the first steps towards feeling better. Remember, no one else is going to see this. Do not use any mental filters and don't let your logical mind take over. Let your thoughts flow. Afterwards, tear this up and throw it away. (If you are using a laptop or a phone, do not save it.)

If you find yourself crying, let the tears flow.

When we identify and acknowledge our emotions, we are accepting reality for what it is. Instead of avoiding it, we are giving an outlet to our emotions so that they do not fester and grow inside us. This lifts the pressure of 'always look on the bright side'. Sometimes there simply is no bright side, and that is okay!

In Julia Cameron's book *The Artist's Way*, which is essentially a twelve-week course for creative people who are feeling stuck, she talks about a technique called 'The Morning Pages'. She recommends keeping a journal and recording all our thoughts. She asks us to fill three pages without stopping to think. She says that if we have nothing to write we could simply write 'I have nothing to write' repeatedly till the mandatory three pages are filled. She says by 'emptying' our mind of thoughts, it makes way for new thoughts.

I have tried this exercise for weeks, and I was astounded at the wisdom that emerged after a few days. A lot of people report the same thing, that they have immensely benefitted from 'releasing' their thoughts. Pushing back against a strong emotion might make it build up inside us. But when we express it, it is like a 'safety valve'.

Use your safety valve as often as you like.

2. Change

Once we have identified and expressed our primary emotion, we are ready to take the next step towards the magic mindset. This is to bring about a change in how we currently feel.

A. Change location

The easiest way to bring about a shift in the energy is to change our surroundings. Physically remove yourself from the space you are currently in; go for a walk outside, if you can. Leave your phone behind, so that you are not tempted to check messages to distract yourself from your thoughts. As you walk, think about what you have expressed. Allow it to flow through your mind. Walk briskly and inhale deeply. Walk till you feel better. Then return.

Physical activity is also a powerful mood elevator. A study conducted by the Harvard School of Public Health shows that running for fifteen minutes a day or walking for an hour daily reduces the risk of major depression by 26 per cent. Exercise calms our mind. It stimulates our body to release the feel-good endorphins. Science also tells us that physical activity increases the activity in the hippocampal neurons, which store memories and increase our ability to process old and new memories, keeping them distinct and separate.

Whenever I have been extremely upset about something I cannot change, I cycle to a lake nearby. Being outdoors and inhaling fresh air calms my mind, and I come back in a better frame of mind, ready to tackle whatever surprise life may throw at me.

B. Change the atmosphere

Changing the atmosphere in our room can also help immensely. Ever noticed how even a simple act like changing the position of the furniture or adding a new piece suddenly makes the place look fresh and different? The ancient Chinese system of feng shui relies on the placement of things in the 'right place' to create a harmonious flow of energy.

Whether you believe in feng shui or not, reorganizing your furniture can bring a breath of freshness to your space. If you do not want to rearrange furniture or are limited by space constraints, even a simple act such as changing your bed covers and pillow covers can help! You could also tidy your wardrobe if you feel like it. Many of my friends swear by this and vouch for the sense of control it gives them.

Clear the clutter: Clearing clutter is a personal favourite of mine. Having read Marie Kondo's *Life-Changing Magic of Tidying Up* and having practised what she suggests, I can vouch that her methods truly work. While her system is time consuming and will take several weeks or days, we can incorporate some of what she advocates to improve our lives, especially the bit about keeping only those things that 'spark joy'.

Look around your room or home and choose the messiest area you have been neglecting. It could be your terrace or your wardrobe or the kitchen sink. Begin by cleaning or tidying one small bit of it, if you do not have the time or energy to do it fully. In your wardrobe, it could be a single shelf. If it's your desk, you could tidy a single drawer. It can even be a simple thing like making your kitchen sink shine or simpler still, perhaps stitching a button that came off or fixing a squeaky door hinge by applying oil. Perhaps it is your bookshelf that needs tidying? Or maybe there is too much dust that has gathered on your TV cabinet. Look around your home, choose one area that needs a shine, get your cleaning supplies and get to work!

Some people mistake clearing clutter with being minimalist and throwing out everything they have spent good money on. I don't believe in that. What I mean by clearing clutter is going through the contents of my desk or wardrobe or kitchen and giving away things that I no longer use or throwing away things that are broken. This helps in changing the general atmosphere, and whenever I have done this, I have always felt better.

Rely on music: Brain researchers have found that listening to music that we love causes a dopamine surge in our bodies—the same feel-good chemical that is released when we fall in love, have sex or eat food rich in salt. Powerful music evokes the deepest of emotions in us, which explains why so many people cry after listening to an opera piece, even when they don't understand the language. Music is also a quick and effective way to change our state of mind.

A few years back, Dr Shyam Bhatt, a psychiatrist and integrative medicine specialist, launched one of my books. The book was about unrequited love and the deep grief that comes with a relationship not working out. While we conversed about many things, one of the things that stuck in my head is the method he recommended to the audience to feel better about a situation one felt helpless and sad about. He said an effective way would be to choose three songs—

the first could be a sad song that expresses how we feel; the second should be a slightly happier song; the third one should be a peppy upbeat number. By the third song, our mood is certain to have changed!

Use candles or aroma dispensers: My bedside cabinet always has a few candles, an essential oil dispenser and incense. I find them to be great for improving my mood. The candles are mostly gifts from my friends and my personal favourite is one from a dear friend—a White Barn scented candle called Paris Cafe, which smells of coffee when lit.

When I lived in Pondicherry, I discovered products from Auroville and fell in love with them. One of their products is an organic natural incense that does not emit harmful chemicals. I have stocked up on the scents I love—patchouli, jasmine, musk. Recently I discovered an NGO called Antarkranti, which sells incense made by the inmates in Indian prisons. I felt it was a good cause to support, as it is a means of livelihood for the inmates who can be rehabilitated and reintegrated into the society if they have a source of income.

Aromatherapy is a fast and effective way to change the way I feel. There is something calming about a familiar, well-loved fragrance. Experiment and try out different fragrances and see which ones you like and then keep them handy for bleaker moments in life.

Indulge in flowers: I love having fresh flowers around me. They instantly brighten up any place and make it look festive. Perhaps you could walk to the florist and come back with a bunch of your favourite flowers. This allows you to get some exercise and buy something to brighten your room. If you want the flowers to last long, make a vertical cut on the stem, before you place them in water. Continue trimming the stem every two days with vertical cuts and change the water every day to make the blooms last longer.

You could gift yourself a flower subscription box and get fresh flowers on a certain day of the week. If your city has no flower subscription services, you could work out a deal with the florist. You do not have to buy expensive flowers; even a small bunch of seasonal flowers will do the job.

C. Practise acts of kindness

To feel better about something, practise small acts of kindness. You could make a small donation to your favourite charity; buy a small gift for a friend; allow someone to go ahead of you in a line at the supermarket; pay for the coffee of the person behind you at a coffee shop; volunteer to spend time reading to the elderly at a home—the possibilities are endless.

If you do not want to do any of these or are unable to, you could simply smile and wish the people you pass by when you walk. In other words, spread some kindness and happiness. It is sure to make you feel good and put a smile on the face of the recipient.

3. Detach, Don't Dwell

We all live under the illusion that we have control over our outcomes, stemming from the conditioning that tells us that if we do our bit, we will get everything we strive for. But in truth, we don't control *anything*, or at least very little that matters.

Here's a little experiment. Speak to ten people you know. Ask them if they are in the career they always hoped for or whether they made a switch because they realized what they were doing was making them unhappy. Chances are, seven of them will tell you they switched careers or that they are in a career they never even thought they would be in.

Life often sends us down tunnels we never anticipated. We must empower ourselves to dig our way out of them and emerge stronger. Sometimes, the path we have chosen gets rocky. Sometimes we might come across a situation where there is simply no road ahead. When it seems like we are up against an insurmountable wall, what can we do?

The Inspiring Story of Zachary Moore

I find the story of Zachary Moore very inspiring. Zachary went from serving a prison sentence for murder to a $100K+ engineering job. For twenty-two years, Zachary lived in a 6x9 prison cell. Today, he sits in an open-plan office in San Francisco, working as a coder. Zachary grew up with domestic abuse, as both his parents were alcoholics. Sharing feelings was discouraged, and as a teenager, he had trouble managing his emotions. He used drugs and alcohol to cope. In 1996, after a distressing argument with his family, his years of misplaced rage, anger, jealousy and pain exploded, pushing Zachary over the edge, and he stabbed his sibling to death. In 1997, he was sentenced to twenty-six years of life imprisonment. For the next few years, Zachary was shunted from prison to prison, and he grappled with who he was and what he had done. Prison was hell; he had to deal with older men, hardened criminals. He began getting into frequent bouts of trouble for misconduct. In 2000, he was thrown into 'Ad-seg for serious misconduct'. 'Ad-seg' is also called 'the hole', and the prisoners are locked in their cells for twenty-three hours a day, with very little human contact.

It was here that he began his journey inwards, where he began 'peeling the layers' and accepting the things he needed to address and fix. He had always struggled with extreme anxiety and he now needed to make psychological changes if he wanted to change his life. He gravitated towards a group of men who were trying to better themselves. Though they were bullied and ridiculed by others, they formed a 'brotherhood' of sorts and began supporting each other emotionally. Zachary began attending Buddhist services. Meditation taught him techniques to cope with his anxiety. He learnt to recognize what he was feeling, and that it was okay to feel that way. Breathing techniques grounded him, and he learnt to cope with his mind over a period of time. In 2010, when Silicon Valley entrepreneur Chris Redlitz was invited to give a business talk to inmates at San Quentin Prison, he expected to 'find a bunch of bad people' but after he gave the talk, he realized they were skilled entrepreneurs who had no avenue to express themselves. He founded 'The Last Mile' to empower inmates with hireable skills, so that the cycle of crime could be broken.[12] Zachary applied for the programme started by The Last Mile, and there, he learnt that failure was

---

12 Seven out of ten released inmates commit a crime within three years as they have no job, housing or skills.

temporary. He learnt to work in a group, towards a common goal. The sense of achievement he felt when he coded and built something was immense. Zachary said though there was the heavy feeling of dread that he would never ever walk out of prison, he learnt to detach himself from that feeling when he coded. He did not dwell on what he could not change or control, and immersed himself in the task at hand.

Like Zachary, we must learn to 'switch off' and focus only on the things we can control. If your situation or surroundings overwhelm you, withdraw from it for a while. Do something different from your usual routine. It could be something as simple as taking a barefoot walk on the grass or trying out a new recipe. You could also rekindle a hobby you have been neglecting. Do something small that gives you joy.

We need to regularly rest our thoughts and minds, and park our gloom and pessimism. This can help us to not dwell on things we feel helpless about. Once we have put in all our effort towards fulfilling our desired outcomes, we must let it go and hope for the best. If things don't go our way, perhaps that wasn't the plan the universe had for us. Something better is in store.

4. Create Peace

When I mention the word meditation, a common reaction from younger people is, 'Ew, mediation is for oldies', or 'Meditation is boring'. Some try it and find it difficult. Some give up because they are unable to control their thoughts.

Years ago, when I was a teen, my father taught me meditation. I found it hard to sit still, but he guided me through it. His voice was deep, almost hypnotic. He would have me imagine a lake with placid waters and a bright blue sky with white fluffy clouds; he would then ask me to imagine a pebble or a stone falling into the clam waters. He would tell me to picture the ripples and ask me to visualize how they spread and then slowly died down till the water became calm again. With my father speaking, I was able to do this. At first, my thoughts kept wandering but with practice, I got used to sitting still and became better at it.

Later, my father would tell me to visualize my problem and 'put it into the stone', which then sank to the bottom of the lake. It helped me be in a better frame of mind and after the meditation, whatever problem I had, didn't seem so 'big' any more. What he had been teaching me was a visualization technique, an exercise that helped me to 'create my peace'.

But once I got married and got busy with two children, running a home and working, I forgot all about meditation. There simply was no time to sit in peace and meditate, with the demands of two young kids. When my children became slightly older and started school, I did have time to myself, but didn't see any need to set aside time for meditation. It was limited to a few moments of closing my eyes, in my yoga class, after which I went about my daily life.

A few years ago, I was hit by a bout of insomnia. No matter what I tried, I simply couldn't sleep. I got a complete health check-up done and there really were no underlying medical issues. Though the doctors suggested an herbal sleeping aid, I was reluctant to take it. That was when a friend suggested meditation, along with breathing exercises. She volunteered to teach it to me. I began meditating again after many years, along with breathing exercises—religiously setting aside time for it. In a few weeks, my insomnia disappeared.

Our mind is a vortex of thoughts and emotions. While some studies say that we have over 12,000 thoughts a day, others say we have about 6,000. One study claims that 85 per cent of the thoughts we have are negative. The exact number of thoughts does not matter; what does is that our mind is a very busy place.

Once we begin thinking, we simply cannot stop. We fall into 'thought loops', often unaware of it. For instance, you might think of a presentation that is due tomorrow, and then you might remember that your boss asked you to look into that pending issue, which reminds you that the colleague who said they would get back to you on it didn't and then you remember the instances where this colleague has done it several times in the past, you wonder how people can be so irresponsible and—well, you get the picture. The thoughts spiral and go on and on. They go on inside our heads when we eat, shower, walk, cook or do household chores. They go on, whether we are alone or whether you have company. Even when we watch an engrossing TV show, the brain is processing and trying to make connections between our life and whatever we are watching on screen. There simply is no respite from thoughts.

One way of stopping these thought loops is to become conscious of them. The mind can be trained. Meditation is a simple and powerful technique that you can use to create your own oasis of peace, especially when you cannot do anything to change the situation you find yourself in.

If you have never meditated before, do not worry. It is easier than you think.

Guided Meditation:

1. Tell the people you are living with that you do not wish to be disturbed for twenty minutes.
2. Grab a good pair of headphones. If you have noise-cancelling headphones, I highly recommend them.
3. Loosen any tight clothing you are wearing. Adjust the fan or the air conditioner or the heater. You must be comfortable.
4. On YouTube search for 'five-minute guided meditation'. There are many guided meditations available. Some are for stress relief. Some are for positive thinking and energy. Choose any that appeals to you. I personally like the meditations by The Honest Guys. Whatever you choose, make sure you find the voice in the guided meditation calming and soothing. If you do not like the voice or if the one you have chosen doesn't work for you, then just pick another.
5. Practise this guided meditation daily. Once you do this for about two weeks, increase the duration. You can now choose a ten-minute guided meditation. You will soon reach a point where you fall asleep. You are training your body and mind to relax and be in the moment.
6. After you get used to the guided meditation, you are now ready to start regular mediation.

Regular Meditation:

1. Download a mediation app that will mind the time for you. Set it to three minutes.

2. Now sit in a comfortable position, close your eyes and focus on your breath.
3. It doesn't matter if your thoughts wander. Allow them to flow. Every time your mind wanders, bring it back to your breath. Don't worry about your mind's endless chatter in the background. Simply remind yourself to be aware of your breath.
4. Do this every day and increase the time duration gradually. When three minutes becomes easy, change the timer to six minutes and so on.
5. If you like, you can keep a meditation journal next to you, and after you open your eyes, you could record the 'insights' or 'wisdom' that came to you. I have been meditating for a few years now, and I can sit in silence for up to 30 minutes. The insights I get after each session continue to astound me.

Science has proven numerous neurological benefits of mediation. MRI scans show the changes in brain activity when one meditates. It produces measurable changes in the brain; reduces anxiety and depression; and improves concentration, attention span and over all psychological well-being. All it takes is ten minutes of our time and costs us nothing!

So why not give this amazing practice a try? Meditation has changed my life. It is not as mysterious or difficult as it seems and helps centre our thoughts and emotions, taking us to a dimension we never thought possible. If you already practise meditation, I am sure you will agree with everything I have said above.

The practice of ACDC is also something I have been doing for many years now. While it doesn't change reality, over which we have no power anyway, it does help us to face it and manage it better.

Try to adopt all these practices for ten days. Make a commitment to stick to it for just that long as a small first step. It is hard to commit for a month, but when we break down our goals into smaller units of time, and then stick to it, a sense of accomplishment goads us on towards our next milestone. You are certain to see a visible change in your mood and your approach to things by following these. Once you have followed it for ten days, you could extend the time period till it becomes a habit, a way of life, a *magic mindset* that greatly improves your quality of life.

The Magic Mindset for Situations Beyond Control

Principle 1: Accept the Feelings
Principle 2: Take Baby Steps

Practice ACDC

1. Acknowledge
2. Change
a) Change the location
b) Change the atmosphere
    - Clear the clutter
    - Rely on music
    - Use candles and aroma dispensers
    - Indulge in flowers
c) Practise acts of kindness
3. Detach, Don't Dwell
4. Create Peace

10
Magic Mindset for Haunting Memories

Memories are bullets. Some whiz by and only spook you. Others tear you open and leave you in pieces.
—Richard Kadrey

I RECEIVED A MAIL FROM ONE OF MY READERS (LET'S CALL her Akshita) in her mid-twenties. She has a job at a PR agency. According to Akshita, she is fairly well adjusted, cheerful and easy to get along with, but she has a difficult boss. No matter what she does, her boss is never satisfied and constantly takes digs at her and demeans her work. Akshita says that once she gets home, whatever happened that day at work keeps playing inside her head. She simply isn't able to let it go. She bristles at the indignation she suffers. She wants to stand up to her boss and express that she is being treated unfairly. After each incident, Akshita thinks about what happened at work and comes up with different ways in which she could have responded. But each time it actually happens, she keeps quiet and puts up with the humiliation. She needs the job since it is a well-paying one, and though she has looked for alternatives, she isn't able to find one. She feels stuck. She in unhappy and upset, unable to get over the memories of the cruel jibes she faces every day.

Another reader (let's call him Pratyush) wrote to me telling me that he finds it hard to let go of the girl he was deeply in love with. They had a three-year relationship, and they dreamt of a future together. But her parents objected strongly to their relationship. In the end, she broke up with him and got married to a guy her parents chose. She has moved on and has a child now who is two and a half. But Pratyush is unable to get over her. He is unable to stop the memories of his time with her and feels stuck.

Memories Make Us Who We Are

In the movie *Eternal Sunshine of the Spotless Mind*, a romantic science-fiction movie, the protagonists Joel and Clementine undergo a scientific process to erase their memories. They meet after their memories have been erased and feel deeply drawn to each other, not knowing how intense their relationship used to be. The narrative shifts to Joel's mind during the memory-erasing procedure. As the procedure progresses, Joel realizes that he doesn't want to erase the memories at all.

Memories are what make us the person we are today. Without our memories, our past becomes a clean slate, and the people who were important in our past cease to matter. Those suffering from advanced Alzheimer's don't even recognize their loved ones—a painful experience for everyone involved.

Every single action we take in our current life is because of our memories, which have given us the lessons we have retained. We grow as we draw wisdom from our experiences. Whatever we go through in life changes us in some way. Whether the memories are painful or pleasant, they trigger growth in us. But sometimes, like Akshita or Pratyush, we get stuck on certain memories. We aren't able to get over a particular incident or a particular time in our lives. We keep playing the incidents on a loop inside our heads, unable to let go.

While Akshita's and Pratyush's cases could be extremes, we are all affected to some extent by our memories. We've all faced situations where something that someone said has hit us in the gut, and we remember it even many years later. We're also familiar with situations where someone cracked a joke at our expense, but we couldn't come up with a quick repartee right then. Much later, we keep thinking about what we could have done and said, but at that moment, we were like a deer caught in headlights.

Memories can haunt us with regret over something we did or said—or didn't. Maybe someone in the family is in a situation where we cannot really do anything and yet watching them in pain makes us unhappy, and we get caught in the rut of obsessing about it. If we keep replaying unhappy memories over and over, and are unable to stop, it becomes unhealthy.

The Problems of Obsessing over Memories

1. Gets Us Stuck in a Problem Rut

When we are obsessively thinking about a situation and wondering why in the world something tragic happened the way it did, we get stuck in the 'problem rut'. We keep lamenting about it, without really moving forward. Akshita and Pratyush are trapped in this 'problem' zone to the extent where they are paralysed, unable to snap out, tormented by the memories.

In the TV series *Lucifer,* hell is depicted as the thoughts that play continually on a loop. It is the person's most shameful and embarrassing thought, the moment they feel most guilty about, that is replayed in their heads. They are trapped in a hell of their own making. They have to keep experiencing the agony of the worst incident from their lifetime—an incident that is in the past but is made real in the present by their minds. Thus, they relive that unhappy memory over and over, suffering terribly. When we rehash our painful memories, we are doing the same.

What is interesting to note is when something good happens, we never ponder over it. We are jubilant and we accept our good fortunes. We don't keep thinking, 'Why did we get so lucky?'

By constantly thinking about a situation we cannot change, or the way a person behaved, we are putting a block in our own 'energy field.' Visualize a stream in full flow. If someone places a rock or a slab of granite in the middle of the stream, its path is blocked. The stream now either splits up into two and flows around the rock or slab, or it completely changes direction. The stream doesn't get stuck. With constant practise, we can train our mind to be like this stream of water. We do not have to get stuck in circumstances that happened to us in the past. There is a way to break free of our thoughts.

2. Creates a Pity Party Loop that Doesn't Get Us Anywhere

When we keep lamenting about a situation, we're essentially throwing ourselves a pity party. We are so hurt by the situation that we want an outlet. We want to be heard. We want someone to acknowledge how terrible our situation is. That isn't a bad thing at all. But if we become trapped in this cycle, then we begin to believe we are truly helpless.

We are allowed to vent about how sad our life is, how cruel fate has been to us and how we do not deserve any of what has happened to us. But we must remember to put a stop to it. The friend who has lent a willing ear leaves with a few kind words. What we forget is that the friend gets on with their life. But in our heads, the pity party continues. Many of us find it hard to break out of this cycle, because our reality is what it is! Things *are* bad. We cannot pretend they aren't. Talking to our friends about it brings us some relief. Thus, we continue.

My grandmother was one of the most stoic women I knew. She was married at eleven. Child marriages were common, back then. Throughout her lifetime, she faced many hardships. She had five children and often there wasn't enough food, but together with my grandfather, she managed to raise them. Both my grandparents had a policy they adhered to all their lives: never complain. My grandmother said that if we have many shoulders to cry on, we will cry more. She told us if we cannot do anything about a situation, we just have to put up with it, and carry on. 'Crying about it gets you nowhere, so you might as well laugh,' she used to say. My grandmother was extremely cheerful and had a laugh that was infectious. I have no idea how she managed to do it, but the lesson she imparted has remained with me.

3. Distracts Us from Current Goals

As a writer, I visit many places in my head I would rather not go to. I have to dredge up old memories, examine them and see if they make good material for the scene I am writing. If I get stuck in an old memory, I have trained my mind to snap out of it. If I do not do that, it becomes hard for me to write further. I have learnt to compartmentalize things inside my head and put a tight lid on past memories. After I examine a memory, I have to put it away. I do this by taking a break from my writing. I make myself a cup of tea and I spend time in my garden or watch fifteen minutes of my current TV series. If I don't do that, I get lost in the memory maze, and it distracts me from the goal at hand, which is to complete my book.

When we keep thinking about something, we are taking ourselves farther away from our goals. The more we obsess, the harder it becomes to go forward towards our destination. These memory bylanes are tricky and best avoided. If at all we have to visit them, we should do so but quickly get back to the present reality. Don't be trapped in the annals of the past.

4. Harms Our Well-being

Obsessive thinking and lamenting get us down. It harms our overall mental well-being. It can affect our confidence as all our present actions are coloured by the events that happened in the past. Pratyush is unable to form a relationship with anyone as he keeps thinking about the unfairness of the treatment he received. Akshita is not able to stand up for herself because she sees herself as a victim. The constant chatter in her head tells her she is being picked on and the incidents that happen reiterate this belief.

I love this quote by the Greek philosopher Heracltius: 'A man cannot step into the same river twice. It is not the same river, and it is not the same man.' What it means is that we are continuously changing, and so are our circumstances. When an incident happens to us first, we are different. We then evolve into a different person than we used to be. Yet our behaviour is controlled by our memories. Staying trapped in those thoughts ruins a perfectly good present.

Are there ways to break out of the trap of the past? What if a situation is so terrible that it feels like there's no hope at all? What if someone close to us is terminally ill? What if we are stuck in a terrible relationship but there is no way out of it? What if the behaviour of a family member hurts us, and despite communicating several times, they continue to act in selfish ways? What if we have a boss like Akshita's or a past relationship like Pratyush's?

Exercise 9a

If you are tormented by a particular memory of an incident that happened in the past, write it down.

Exercise 9b

Write down this affirmation: 'I did my best at that time, in the manner I was capable of. That version of me no longer exists. I let go of that version of me. I forgive myself.'

After you have written down the affirmation above, you have 'released' the memory.

You can now *choose* to act in a way that is more beneficial to your mental well-being.

Rather than being victims of our thoughts, we can take concrete actions that make us feel better. Even if we cannot change the situation, we can change the way we look at it. Even in the most difficult of circumstances, we can do certain things to help us cope better.

With constant practise, we can train our minds to think in a certain way. Just like the stream that changes its course when an obstacle appears, we *can* carve an alternate path for ourselves. We do not have to be trapped by our pasts. We can liberate ourselves from destructive thought patterns that hold us back.

Principle 1: Redefine Yourself

Many years ago, I found myself at a very negative place. I had been very unfairly treated, professionally. I put everything I had into a project I was assigned. I rearranged my schedule several times to accommodate all the requests made by my employers. I sacrificed several personal commitments that meant a lot to me. At the very last minute, the big project that I had worked on was dropped. The people I was dealing with gave me a very flimsy excuse, and no explanations whatsoever. It cost me my mental peace. I was constantly thinking about how shabbily I had been treated. My contract was such that I couldn't quit or avoid further professional commitments. Despite being treated like dirt, I had to continue to deliver.

For a couple of weeks, I was cursing my employers. It began seeping into other areas of my life. My irritability rose, and I was taking it out on people who had nothing to do with it. After a few weeks, I was tired of being stuck in this terrible place. I decided I had had enough and resolved to help myself.

We are victims of our own thoughts and the only way we can stop being a victim is if we create a new version of ourselves.

Principle 2: Be a Fighter, Not a Victim

When I decided that I no longer wanted to be controlled by my memory of how I was treated by my employers, I followed a technique that involved four simple steps. I have now named it the RISE technique.

The next time you get stuck in bad memories, you can use these four steps to get out of them.

1. Recognize

The first step is to *recognize* and be aware of when you begin to obsess. The typical obsessive thought might start when there's a trigger. (Someone saying something or doing something, or something we see). We then go into a loop of unwanted thoughts. For me, this was when I saw anything related to a company with which I had a professional commitment. When I saw an ad by them or a social media post, the negative thoughts would begin. The first step was to be aware.

The next time this happens, make an attempt to recognize what you are doing. Be conscious of your thoughts. If the thoughts are obsessive and strong, start making a note of them in your phone, laptop or a journal. Call this the 'thought journal' and start writing the thoughts that are going on inside your head along with the time and date. It could be something like this:

I have texted my friend, and I keep checking the phone every two minutes to see if she has responded.

Or

I am angry at _____ because he doesn't care about how he makes me feel. I feel like he does it deliberately to hurt me.

Or

I think I looked like a fool when I responded this way to _____. How stupid will he think I am.

Or

I am so angry at how they have treated me, I am bristling with rage. My fists are clenched, and I am breathing shallower.

Or

_____ has been so mean, rude and unkind to me. I don't think she deserves me as a sibling.

Or

I never treat him this way, then why does he do this to me?

Once these thoughts are out in the open and have taken a concrete shape through words, it becomes easier to identify a pattern as well as the trigger. You will figure out how many times a day you think of this and find that writing it out gets it 'out of your head' and gives you some relief, even if it is temporarily.

2. Interfere

It is very important to *interfere* with these thoughts. The first step towards this is writing down the thoughts in the thought journal. Then, read what you have written. Use a timer and give yourself about ten minutes (or lesser) to think about everything you have written. Allow yourself to be immersed in pity, grief, anger or sorrow—or anything that you feel when you read the thoughts. When the timer goes off, STOP. Tell yourself that the pity party or the anger party is over. You now have to leave.

Remember, what is written are just thoughts. They exist only inside your head and on the paper. They are a bunch of neurons firing off messages to our brain cells. Let them exist there. Do not fight them. Do not try to change them. Accept them. These thoughts are not the current reality. They are in the past and have made you feel a certain way. But that is not your reality in the moment. You're simply reliving your pain or shame or embarrassment from the past. You are a different person now. Tell yourself that you can live with these thoughts. You do not have to do anything about them for now. It is enough to just be aware, write them down, and then STOP. If you do nothing about them, they will just pass. They are fleeting.

Once you start recording these thoughts and allowing them to exist, you will notice that the frequency of these thoughts has reduced. The time gap between the obsessive thoughts will increase gradually.

3. Write Down All the Solutions

Once you have done the above exercises a few times, you will discover that you have put a distance between yourself and your thoughts. You are now able to separate your emotions from the event that has happened. In case you are still not able to do that, go back and repeat step two for a few more days or a few more weeks.

Training our mind takes time and practice. Patterns of thoughts are something we have lived with for years. They are not going to vanish like magic just because we do the exercise once. Accept that it is going to take time. Do it over and over. Notice how you learn to recognize and interfere every time you have a 'memory attack'.

When you become adept at separating the emotions from the incident that has occurred in the past, examine the problem like an outsider. Perhaps you can create a character who has the same problems that you face. As a novelist, when I create characters, create their personalities, give them problems and allow them to interact, I find that the characters solve their own problems. It is not a conscious process I follow.

By putting distance between you and your problems, and thinking about yourself in the third person, by treating YOU as a character in the story of your life, by removing the immediate emotion, you will perhaps come up with a creative solution.

Write down ALL the solutions you can think of—both probable and improbable. Write it in the third person. Writing in third person tricks your brain into removing emotions and adding objectivity.

For instance:

Akshita can confront her boss and tell her she will take no more.

Or

Akshita can point out all the successful things she did.

Or

Akshita can speak to an experienced friend and seek her advice.

Once you examine the above solutions, you will be in a position to do the best thing. Perhaps you will decide that to do nothing is the best option. Perhaps you will choose to act on one of the things you wrote down to change the situation. It is even possible that once it is off your chest, having thought about it in detail, you will learn to let it go.

4. Empty the Mind

Sit in silence for a few minutes. Practice meditation. (See the previous chapter for mediation techniques.) Practice mindfulness. Focus on breathing, and as you sit in silence, observe your breath. Allow the thoughts to come and go. Become aware that they are like clouds. Sometimes, they will be dark and come loaded with rain. Once it pours, they will leave. Sometimes they will be soft and fluffy, and they will slowly float away.

The thing to be most aware of is that thoughts will come and just as they come in, they will go too. Allow them to enter and exit. You don't have to act on anything. What you are doing is fighting the memories by offering no resistance, and with time, their power over you will vanish. The next time you are continually thinking about something that happened in the past, try to RISE above it by following all the steps mentioned above.

Magic Mindset for Haunting Memories

Principle 1: Redefine Yourself
Principle 2: Be a Fighter, Not a Victim

The Problems of Obsessing over Memories:

1. Gets Us Stuck in a Problem Rut
2. Creates a Pity Party Loop that Doesn't Get Us Anywhere
3. Distracts Us from Current Goals
4. Harms Our Well-being

To stop letting memories dictate our lives, we must RISE:

1. Recognize
2. Interfere
3. Write Down All the Solutions
4. Empty the Mind

11
Magic Mindset for Exams and Interviews

Hannah Abbott became the first to receive a Calming Draught from Madam Pomfrey after she burst into tears during Herbology and sobbed that she was too stupid to take exams and wanted to leave school now.
—J.K. Rowling

W E'VE ALL FACED THIS AT SOME POINT OR THE OTHER in our lives. We study hard and practise a lot for an interview or an exam. When we are by ourselves, we seem to know everything. Though we are a little apprehensive, we're fairly sure we will do well. Then it happens. When the question paper is thrust in front of us, there is that moment of panic. Our heart thuds in our ears. Our palms become sweaty. An insane fear grips us, throwing all logic and reasoning out of the window. We make errors even though we had practised, and this fuels the fear. If we are being interviewed, our palms grow cold. We say things we never intended to. If it's an interview where we have to solve actual problems while the interviewers watch, it is even more stressful.

I am yet to meet a person who has not faced any or all of the above at some point in their lives. It is only normal to get stressed. We are stressed because how we perform matters to us. We want to excel. We want to do our best—and that is a good thing, is it not?

While it may not be possible to get rid of the stress entirely, we could take some steps to manage it, and work it to our advantage.

Principle 1: Preparation Is Most of the Battle Won

Facing an important exam or an interview is like going to war. We have to prepare for it for months in advance or at least weeks or days in advance. When I was a student, I experienced terrible exam anxiety. I was a good student, and topped almost every exam I took, but that didn't help me be less nervous. I was terrified of performing badly. Over the years, I developed my own coping mechanisms.

1. Prepare Well

The first step, of course, is to prepare—and prepare well. This might seem like an obvious one, but you'd be surprised how many people turn up unprepared or inadequately prepared, which increases their nervousness.

When I was in school, I was selected to play for the KVS Nationals in basketball. It was a big deal, as the team had to travel to different states to compete with others. This also involved missing a lot of classes. Long hours of practice often meant I was too tired to be alert during class time. But I made up for it at home by preparing hard. I stuck a yearly planner on my wall. The first thing I did was write the dates of the exams. This showed me the time I had left till D-day. Then I broke down subjects to be studied, lesson wise. After this, I allocated the chapters to each day. For example, Monday: Mathematics, Chapter 1 to 3. This way, I knew exactly what I would be studying on a certain day. I planned it out in such a way that by the time of the exam, I would have completed studying the portion and revised it well. The planner that I stuck on my wall helped me allocate my time wisely. It gave me small achievable goals. I felt motivated when I put a tick mark at the end of the day, where I had accomplished what was planned. And the best part? It was all right in front of me—at a glance, I could see my progress and what needed to be done further. This helped me alleviate that 'out-of-control' feeling to a great extent, as I knew I was adequately prepared.

If you know the date of the exams, plan well in advance. Breaking down the biggest tasks into smaller manageable chunks goes a long way.

2. A Tip to Assimilate Information—Taking Breaks

Preparation is only effective if we allow the brain the time and space to relax so that the knowledge is absorbed and retained. Relaxation is a big part of this. This is something I follow to this day, say, when I am working on a book. Working on a book is a long-term activity that requires months of dedication and discipline to complete. What helps me is taking breaks where I switch off for a while. I either tend to the garden or cook. Sometimes, I take my cycle and go for a small ride.

You could adapt this while preparing for an exam or interview. Rather than studying for three hours continuously for an exam, study for twenty to thirty minutes. Then take a five-minute break where you do not think about what you studied. This helps you to assimilate the information. It also helps to 'clear your head' and refreshes you. The key here is not to get distracted from your goal during the break. Don't let the five-minute break extend to fifteen minutes because your attention has been diverted by a reel on Instagram or a YouTube video. If you can, go outdoors and walk for five minutes. Leave your phone at home. Then get back. If you live in an apartment complex, you can walk around the building. Not only will those small walks help you stay focused but will also add to your fitness.

Principle 2: Look Back at How Far You've Come

1. See the Big Picture

Many a time when we take an exam or appear for an interview, we're not focused on our long-term goals. The only thing looming before us is the immediate task on hand, which is the exam or the interview. All our energies are directed towards clearing this one hurdle and we forget the big picture. We ignore how it will be five years from now or ten years from now and don't give ourselves enough credit for the progress we have made.

Try and remind yourself of your whole life. Look at how far you have come from where you were before. Look back at the road you have travelled. Perhaps five years ago, even giving this exam/interview would have been just a dream for you. Pause. Look back. In two years from now, you will be even farther ahead on that road. This trial will only be a small dot on your timeline. In case this doesn't go well, there will always be another chance. This line of thinking will help to put things into perspective.

2. Sum Up Your Achievements

Exercise 10

You will need about ten to fifteen minutes of undisturbed time for this exercise. Divide your life into sets of five years. Write down every small achievement that you can think of, starting from birth. Put down even the small things you remember. It does not matter whether you consider it a 'big deal' or whether everyone has achieved the same. This is about you and what you have accomplished.

Close your eyes and rest for three minutes (use a timer). Now, open your eyes and read the list. The point of this exercise is to give yourself a morale boost. When you write down all that you have accomplished, you focus on everything that you have done right so far and have succeeded at. This one exam or interview is not going to determine your entire life.

Principle 3: Switch Off and Relax

A day before and on the day of the exam or the interview, there are some steps you can take to ensure you are calm. The fifteen minutes before you take the exam or the time when you are waiting, outside, to be called in for the interview are crucial. It is during this time that stress levels peak, which can affect your performance.

To stay calm on the day of the exam or interview, try the following things that worked for me.

1. Indulge in Distraction

Over the years, I have learnt that the best way to cope with stress is distraction. My school, Kendriya Vidyalaya, was inside the IIT campus in Chennai. The atmosphere was extremely competitive. The parents of most of my classmates were professors at IIT. It was a given that they would all write the IIT entrance exams. Great academic performance was stressed upon.

I wasn't sure what I wanted to do back then. All I knew is that I didn't want anything to do with science. In such an atmosphere, I had to carve out my own niche. This meant putting myself in a protective bubble, where what my classmates did wouldn't affect me much. Before an exam, most people would be furiously turning the pages of the textbook, trying to get some last-minute studying done. I didn't see any point in that. If I hadn't studied for weeks, then nervously flipping through the pages of the textbooks minutes before entering the exam hall would only make me more nervous, especially if I came across things I didn't know. It would shatter my confidence. So I read a novel instead, to take my mind off the exam. Everyone looking at me thought I was either extremely well prepared (I was only reasonably prepared) or that I didn't care. They were wrong. I was doing this to deal with my own stress. And guess what? It helped. I topped most of the exams I took, because I was able to keep my cool and make smarter choices instead of following what others were doing. (Of course it also helped that I had meticulously prepared by studying well in advance.)

Don't be afraid to make a different choice and not conform. Distract yourself to keep your stress levels in check, and don't focus on what is to come while you wait.

2. Watch What You Drink

What we drink before an exam plays a role in how we perform. When we encounter a perceived threat, such as when we are alone, walking down a dark alley or when a menacing dog growls at us on the streets, our hypothalamus (a small region in the brain) sends off a 'high alert' siren. This prompts the adrenal glands, located on top of the kidneys, to release a surge of hormones, including adrenaline and cortisol. Adrenaline increases the heart rate and boosts energy. Cortisol is the stress hormone that increases sugars in the bloodstream and enhances the brain's use of glucose. In other words, our brain is hardwired to prepare us for a 'fight or flight' response. During interviews and exams, we're already 'charged up' with adrenaline and cortisol, so limiting sugar can help us calm our nerves.

Do not have colas (highly loaded in sugar) or fruit juice with added sugar. It's likely to make you more jittery. If you must have coffee, try to have it with no sugar or very little sugar. Drink calming teas like chamomile or good old black tea with mint. A small change in what you drink right before an interview or an exam could go a long way in making you feel calmer.

3. Don't Force Yourself to Calm Down

In one of my favourite movies, *The Shawshank Redemption*, the protagonist, Andy Dufrense, is accused of murdering his wife and her lover, and has to face a hard life in prison—a life sentence. He is bullied and abused and eventually learns to survive the cruelties of prison, which is ruled by hierarchy and a corrupt system. On one occasion, the warden throws Andy in the isolation cell—a dreaded tiny 'hole', where he is cut off from light and all people. It is a feared and severe punishment. Andy later tells his fellow inmates that he was able to survive the hole and keep himself sane by playing Mozart's 'Figaro' in his head.

Though it is a fictional movie, we can take lessons from this. Many prisoners who survived Auschwitz narrate similar incidents. The only thing that gave them the strength to go on was clinging on to happy memories that helped them shut out the miseries of the present. We can use the same techniques to fight stress. Sometimes, when we try too hard to 'be calm', it has the opposite effect. If we are constantly thinking about how stressed we are, we're only going to get more worked up. It also doesn't help if we tell ourselves 'don't get stressed', because we already are.

Instead close your eyes and think of a very happy memory. Go into the memory in vivid detail. Recall the smell, the sights and the sounds. Think about how you felt, who you were with. Think about what was around you. Try to recall every single detail. The deeper you go into the memory, the better. Think about how much fun it was. Allow yourself to daydream about that time for a few minutes. Giving your brain a breather like this allows it to release feel-good hormones that can calm you down. Keep an arsenal of happy memories ready and visit a happy place in your head any time you feel stressed.

4. Breathe

When we are stressed out, breathing is shallow, cutting off essential oxygen to our body cells. Be conscious of how you breathe. If you are getting too stressed while waiting for the interview or the exam to begin, walk away to a secluded spot. Deliberately take slow and deep breaths. Count your breaths as you inhale and exhale. Repeat positive affirmations to yourself:

'Everything will unfold just the way it is meant to be. We don't control anything. May the best manifest.'
Or
'What is more important than the result is the fact that I GET to do this. This is a privilege.'
Or
'All is well, and everything will go well.'

Repeat something that works for you, have a drink of water and go back to the exam hall or the waiting room with renewed confidence and calmness. Remember, a single exam or interview does not make or break anyone. If you fail, there will *always* be other options. Perhaps the universe is guiding you towards a different path. Calm down, do your best and leave the rest. Don't worry about it.

Good luck!

Magic Mindset for Exams and Interviews

Principle 1: Preperation Is Most of the Battle Won
Principle 2: Look Back at How Far You've Come
Principle 3: Switch Off and Relax

Long-term Plan:

1. Prepare Well
2. A Tip to Assimilate Information—Taking Breaks
3. See the Big Picture
4. Sum Up Your Achievements

Immediately Before the Exam/Interview

1. Indulge in Distraction
2. Watch What You Drink
3. Don't Force Yourself to Calm Down
4. Breathe

12

Magic Mindset for Reconciling with Other People's Actions

When you stop expecting people to be perfect, you can like them for who they are.

—Donald Miller

Some time ago, I had put out a quote on my social media on positivity. I suggested that if a situation or person is no longer making us feel good about ourselves, it is time to walk away. In response, I received several messages asking me what to do if the person is a close family member and if we cannot walk away.

One of my young readers told me about how her parents would never see her point of view in anything. Another wrote to me about a toxic mother-in-law who would insist on being a part of everything that she and her husband did. Yet another fifteen-year-old wrote to me about how his family was in debt, and when the debtors would come to their door, he would feel helpless, unable to do anything about it, unable to focus on his exams because of this. A person in her late twenties wrote to me about how she was in love with a certain person who loved her back too, and yet her parents would never accept him as he is of a different caste. Every month, I receive hundreds of variations of the above scenarios where people are stuck in situations, feeling helpless and trapped, affected badly because they are unable to control another person's actions.

Hardwired to Avoid Conflict

If you are born and raised in India (like I was), chances are the ethos that is drilled into you from a very young age tells you to respect your elders, put your family first and to sacrifice your individual needs for the sake of maintaining peace in the family. Without even realizing it, we behave in patterns that avoid confrontation. Right from the clothes we wear to the careers we choose, we are all, to some extent, victims of parental and societal expectations.

I know someone who lives in a very traditional Marwari joint family. The 'rule' is that the daughters-in-laws must wear sarees, with 'ghoonghat'. To 'comply', the son tells his wife to wear a saree in front of his parents but carry western clothes in her bag. Once they leave the house, she changes into western clothes in the restroom of a hotel. The couple then goes out to pubs or bars, and then she changes back into traditional clothes before they return home. I was dumbfounded when I heard this. When I asked her why she and her husband can't stand up to his mother, she said this was the best solution as it avoided conflict.

When I was in college, I had a friend whose parents would not let her get her ears pierced. She used to tell me that she longed to wear pretty earrings like most of us did, but she could wear only plastic 'clip-ons' as her ears weren't pierced. I asked her what would happen if she got her ears pierced and went home. She was terrified at the very thought and said she couldn't do it.

The Burden of Parental Expectations

One of the most common things Indian children are taught is to always obey their parents. But what if what the parents want is very different from what we want for ourselves?

The Netflix reality TV show *Indian Matchmaking*, which made waves internationally, threw a spotlight on how much Indian parents and family control major life decisions. One of the participants, Akshay, is a twenty-five-year-old man from a wealthy family in Delhi. It is his mother who calls the shots about when he should get married, and she is clear that both her sons must obey her. They don't have a choice. They are 'allowed' to choose from the selections that their mother makes. But when it comes to marriage itself, they 'must get married'.

I ran a poll on my Instagram where I asked people in the age group of 22–30 to answer. Over 66 per cent of the respondents said that their parents had broached the topic of their marriage to them and wanted them to get married. When I asked if their parents would be okay if they choose their own life partner, 51 per cent said no. Even in the cases where the parents had left the choice of a life partner to their adult children, many messaged me saying their parents told them that they would be 'happier' if they chose a person from the same caste to fall in love with!

This conflict between our individual needs and what our family wants for us poses a challenge in many areas of life—from major decisions such as marriage to minor ones such as the hairstyle we sport, the friends we make, and at times, even the hobbies we choose. What our family wants for us versus what we want for ourselves is an issue that is hard to deal with. If we keep living according to other people's expectations, it takes a toll on our stress levels. Their advice and suggestions might, no doubt, be well intentioned. They might want the 'best' for us, but their idea of 'what is best' might be completely different from our idea of what is good for us. Very often, families think they know us well, but they don't.

Our families have known us from childhood, and certain patterns of behaviour have been established. Parents might have contributed inadvertently to this. Someone in the family is 'the star', another is 'the troublemaker' and yet another is the 'over-sensitive one'. When we meet after a long time, we are expected to behave a certain way. No matter how much we have changed over the years, and no matter how grown we are, we keep slipping into our childhood roles unless we make a conscious effort to change it. Often, we adopt these roles subconsciously. In families with intense competition between children while growing up, the same conflicts play out when they are adults too. Strangely, it is only with their own families they behave this way. They are perfectly nice individuals, good bosses, model employees and genial to their friends. But when they come back to their families, all of this is erased.

Someone I know told me how much her husband changes when her mother-in-law visits. She says he is a great husband and a good father, but when his mother visits, she sees a side of him (especially with regard to discipling their children) that leaves her shocked. In this case, the mother is the trigger for her husband's behaviour, which in turn affects her badly. She cannot possibly ask her husband to stay away from his mother; she cannot control how he behaves; and she cannot condone this change in his behaviour.

Principle 1: Instead of Trying to Control Others, Control Your Response

We do not have control over how people in our lives—friends, family, colleagues or acquaintances—view the world. However, we do have control over our own emotions and the way we react to others. Over the years, we might have developed our own patterns of behaviour when it comes to dealing with conflicts or remarks by others that hurt us. We may shut them down with a sharp remark; we may give in and feel unhappy about it; or we may ignore them, leading to repeated nagging and unpleasantness. But we can choose to respond differently if the actions of other people affect us.

When we face a situation in which someone's inadvertent remarks or behaviour or expectations puts us in a place of negativity, there are steps we can take to alleviate our distress.

1. Identify the Trigger

Most of the time, we're okay. We are doing our own thing, managing perfectly, and the day looks bright and happy. Then suddenly, someone close to us says something or does something that we don't expect and wham! There's an emotional explosion within us and everything spirals out of control.

Often, the person saying it might not have said it to hurt us. It might be an innocuous remark. Yet, we feel deeply and are hurt or angry or upset. These are called 'emotional' triggers. These are different for different people. A 'trigger' is a situation or a person that makes one react in a disproportional manner, compared to the 'aggression' or the 'crime' or the 'act' committed.

Exercise 11a

If you are affected by other people's behaviour and want to be more in control, write down these details.

1. Where does it happen? (place)
2. When does it usually happen? (time)
3. What happened? (briefly describe the incident)

Some of us are extra sensitive to some things. What is trivial to one person might be a big deal to another. What someone brushes aside as a silly remark might linger on in another's mind for years. We're all products of our conditioning and upbringing. There's no telling which memory might be triggered by an incident.

Right from school, we are conditioned for 'the real world'. We're told to 'be tough' and 'grow up' and 'face life'. Because of societal conditioning and the expectations placed on us, we learn to bury whatever we feel and 'move on' without creating too much of a fuss. Often we rationalize, telling ourselves that we are being too sensitive over a trivial issue. We justify the actions of the other party, excusing them as they didn't mean it in the way they said it.

What we do not acknowledge or delve much into is the reason for our reaction. Why did it hurt us in the first place? Did it create in us a feeling of inadequacy? Did it bring to the forefront our self-doubts, which we thought we had buried deep down? These are issues worth thinking about, if we want to prevent the 'triggers' that make us stressed. The above exercise helps you do that.

2. Be Aware of Your Feelings

Most of the time when someone says something or does something we do not like or approve of, we are *reactive*. We react to what they are saying or doing. Over the years, we develop a pattern of behaviour and often don't even think before responding. We might feel angry, agitated, annoyed, sad, hurt, stressed, upset.

It is important to be aware of what a certain trigger is making us *feel*.

> ## Exercise 11b
>
> When you find yourself reacting emotionally, observe your emotions. Try to define the 'feeling' you are experiencing.
>
> I am feeling_____ because of _____.
>
> Take some time off to *identify* what you feel, as the action unfolds. Is it rage? If so, how angry are you? Is it sadness? If so, why are you feeling sad? If so, what are the reasons for you to feel ashamed?

3. Put Some Distance

To not let a situation spiral out of control, it is important to walk away. But it is equally important to communicate this before walking away. This might be very hard for those who aren't used to standing up for themselves. The other person might get agitated or feel upset that we are shutting them out.

What you tell them is important. You could say, 'This is important to me, and I would like to think about it. I need some time. I will be ready to talk to you after a little while, if you are too.' You have to communicate to the person that you are hurt/upset and you need time to process what happened.

You need to let them know that you aren't 'running away' and instead you need time to think.

Then walk away. If you have your room, go to your room; if not, go out for a walk.

4. Examine

In the privacy of your room (or on a park bench or anywhere where you are alone), sit down with your feelings and examine what you have written down. Acknowledge the feelings, then try to get to the root of the problem. Ask yourself why the person affects you so much. Why do you crave their approval? Why does it matter so much to you, what they said about you or think about you? Why do their actions affect you?

If a stranger was unfair to us, we would probably brush it aside, thinking they are irrelevant because they don't even know us. We'd never give them the importance that you do to a loved one. This is because we have certain expectations from those we love. We presume they will always act in a way that's comfortable for us. We think that our family members or loved ones should listen to us and value our opinion.

Often, we are so hurt that we forget to consider why the person we love behaved in the way they did. Perhaps their behaviour stems from ignorance. Perhaps they are hurting. Perhaps they know no better. Perhaps the choices they make for themselves aren't the ones you would make, and it irks you, because you have no control over their actions or words. Once you get to the 'why', you will be able to process it better.

But this does not mean we have to forgive them instantly. Our feelings of anger, hurt or humiliation are real. If we force ourselves to forgive the person immediately, before we process our emotion, we will end up suppressing that emotion. It will build up inside us, leading to resentment. We are *allowed* to be angry with them or be hurt by their actions.

Remember, all your feelings are *valid*. What is important is to examine where they are coming from.

5. Accept that People Have Their Own Reasons

Conflicts are often a result of expectations. We expect our parents to understand us and be supportive of our decisions. We expect our siblings to be caring, loving and kind towards us. We expect our friends to be there for us, as we would be there for them.

But reality is that at some point, they are going to let us down. We will be disappointed by their behaviour. We cannot control what they say or do. I get mails from my readers where they outline a lot of things that they did for a friend or a loved one, and when they asked for help, the friend or loved one did not reciprocate.

It is possible that the person is selfish. It is also possible that the person is going through something and is not in a place or position to help. For all you know that colleague is jealous of your promotion. Maybe you remind them of something they can never be. Perhaps you have hurt them inadvertently in the past, and they hold it against you. We could spend a long time trying to guess why people behave the way we do. Or we could tell ourselves that people are *allowed* to behave that way because that is who they are in that moment. That is all they are capable of. They are not in a position to give more.

Principle 2: Reclaim Power

By owning our feelings, acknowledging them, waiting for them to settle and then acting, we can take our power back. While we have no control over whether the other person repeats their behaviour or not, we do have control over how we choose to respond. But by putting some distance and thought between the trigger and the subsequent action, we can learn to deal with triggers.

The changes will not happen immediately. They take practice and time, perhaps weeks or months. We must be patient. By taking conscious steps, change is possible. Even if the other person doesn't change, we can, over time, learn to be less affected by their actions, which are not in our control.

1. Decide

After calming down and examining our triggers and emotions, we can decide on the next course of action. The key here is to wait for a couple of days until we are in a better place. In a few days, the situation might change and what is important may not seem so urgent. Every single day, things happen that alter our world view. Time has a way of putting everything in perspective.

If you find yourself still badly hurting after some days have passed, then you should speak to the person about it. It is important that such a conversation is completely calm and most of the feelings of anger or hurt have simmered down. Choose your words carefully and phrase things positively. You could begin by appreciating something that the other person did, and how good it made you feel. You could then bring up the behaviour that hurt you. Take care to phrase it in a manner that states your feelings, rather than emphasize what they did. Do not use an accusatory tone, and never begin a sentence with 'You always ...' unless it is something kind and positive. When we are hurt, the natural instinct is to say 'YOU did this. How could you?' Instead, modify your statements. Calmly narrate what happened and state how it made you feel.

It is important that we take responsibility for our feelings and demand that they be acknowledged, heard and not just brushed aside. Many a time, people are not aware about the impact their actions and words have on others. Chances are the person who caused the hurt is not even aware of how important the issue is for us and how it makes us feel. If our feelings matter to them, and they care deeply, they will make an effort to not repeat their actions.

2. Communicate Assertively

One of the common mistakes we make when we deal with our loved ones is that we presume they should know what we want and do not want, and they should behave accordingly. When a person disappoints us, we either keep quiet (if we are the kind of person who hates a confrontation) and seethe inside or we express our feelings in anger. The other person then picks up on the tone and body language and responds accordingly. Rarely do we communicate in an efficient and assertive manner.

Some of us are masters in disguising our emotions. In *Kim's Convenience*, a Canadian TV series, a Korean convenience store owner in his fifties, Mr Kim, runs the store with his wife. He is an immigrant in Canada, and he now has two adult children. Mr Kim is the epitome of the 'male head of the family'. He rarely displays his emotions and is mostly stoic. Yet, he feels deeply for his family, as is evident in many poignant scenes where he blinks back his tears. Mr Kim is like most of the fathers we know. His daughter, Janet, tries her best to communicate with him, which often ends in exasperation, and she stomps off having failed to get her point across.

Communicating assertively is something you can practise beforehand. If others are used to you communicating in a certain way, you must remember that they may be confused when you speak this way. Pay attention to your body language and tone of voice. Have a pleasant expression and keep your voice soft. Look the other person in the eye and say:

'I need to tell you this and please do hear me out. I've noticed lately that _____.

'This makes me feel _____. We end up _____.

'While I know you are trying to do _____, what it does is, it takes away _____ from me. I go along with you as I am afraid you will get upset. So now on I am going to _____.'

You could modify the above to reflect your unique situation. Assertive communication has to include three things:

1. Understanding the other person's point of view
2. Mentioning the exact problem
3. Telling the person what you want

Exercise 11c

Write down what you are going to say to the person whose behaviour affected you. Begin with a compliment. (It may feel weird to write this down. But it will help you when you speak.) If you aren't used to being assertive, it will take a few tries. Don't give up. Keep emphasizing—gently, kindly and assertively.

While we may not have control over what other people do, following the above steps takes back some of our control over the situation. If we change our approach and modify how we behave and respond to others, we're taking a step in the right direction. The only way to deal with a situation where others behave contrary to our expectations is to be calm and assertive, after assessing what it is that we really want. We are allowed to feel disappointed, but we must train our minds to not be reactive. Bringing about a change is a slow process, and we have to constantly practise the above steps.

Keep trying. Do not give up. And remember, people will not be around forever. Let's accept them with all their faults and shortcomings. When the person is no longer around, what irks us now may make us long for them.

Magic Mindset for Reconciling with Other People's Actions

Principle 1: Instead of Trying to Control Others, Control Your Response
Principle 2: Reclaim Power

Actions to Take

1. Identify the Triggers
2. Be Aware of Your Feelings
3. Put Some Distance
4. Examine
5. Accept that People Have Their Reasons
6. Decide
7. Communicate Assertively

13

The Magic Mindset for Saying No

When dealing with people, remember you are not dealing with creatures of logic, but with creatures bristling with prejudice, and motivated by pride and vanity.

—Dale Carnegie

ONE OF MY READERS EMAILED ME ASKING ME FOR ADVICE on how not to be a 'people pleaser.' When I asked her exactly what she meant, she replied that she knew people were taking advantage of her, but she just couldn't say no. Her query reminded me of a character in a TV series I was watching, who gets taken advantage of all the time. He is a nice person, but his inability to say no makes him do jobs that no one wants to do. He ends up working a lot more than he is paid for, with no weekend time because he is simply unable to say no to a last-minute request from a co-worker.

When I was in my teens, I found it hard to say no to people. I would make excuses so I could avoid the situation I didn't want to be in. Sometimes, I would do whatever was requested of me but feel miserable later. As I entered my twenties, I trained myself to say no by consciously practising it. I read the book *Don't Say Yes When You Want to Say No* by Herbert Fensterheim, and I practised all the exercises the book suggested. Some of the exercises were hard, but I decided to put aside my discomfort and did what was asked.

One of the things I dislike intensely is lending anyone my books. I would earlier lend the books and feel bad when they were never returned. (The one time it was returned, the pages were dog eared and the book had been badly handled.) I decided to put my newly acquired skill of saying no to test, and the next time someone asked me if they could borrow a book from my treasured collection, I said, 'I am really sorry, but I don't lend books.' The person who asked to borrow the books was a relative, so you can imagine my discomfort when I refused. Later, I felt happy about it. I decided that I would rather lose my relationship with the relative than lose the book.

Sometimes, we have no option but to agree to things we do not want to do, especially if we are living with family. For the sake of our family, we might decide to put our personal interests aside and oblige a request that cuts into our time. We do this because we love them and want to do something nice for them. But there is a thin line we tread when we decide to do things for others that we do not want to.

Merriam Webster defines 'people pleaser' as a person who has an emotional need to please others, often at the expense of their own desires. People pleasers say yes to everything that is asked of them.

Psychologists say that saying yes even when we do not want to isn't always bad. It just shows that you are a deeply caring person who values social connections and enjoys making others happy. However, if it is causing you deep inconvenience and you recognize that it is affecting your self-esteem, then you need to stop.

Exercise 12a

Write down instances where you said yes, even though you wanted to say no.

> **Exercise 12b**
>
> How did it make you feel? Did it make you feel resentful or used?

Principle 1: You Have the Right to Say No

When I was in my twenties, I simply never realized that I have the *right* to say no to unreasonable requests. Most of us think 'being nice' is saying yes to whatever is asked of us.

I have a terrible memory associated with one of my book launches many years ago. I must have signed more than fifty copies for readers and was looking forward to spending the rest of the evening with my family and other author friends who had travelled a long way to attend the launch. A book launch is a celebration for readers as well as the author, who spends months and months in isolation while working on the book. At this book launch, a fan kept following me around asking for selfies. Even after signing all the copies he asked me to, he wouldn't leave me alone. I was too naive and too nice to tell him I wanted some privacy as I had obliged *all* his requests. I thought I *owed* him as many pictures as he requested. He must have clicked at least twenty pictures with me. He ruined my evening by following me around everywhere and not letting me even talk to my friends or family. All these years later, all I remember is how terrible I felt to be hounded like that. Now, I am much more assertive and can tell people when I would like to be left alone after I have signed all their copies and posed for selfies with them.

Remember, whenever you say yes to an unreasonable request, you are saying no to yourself and what you really want. You do have a right to say no to people. If you don't exercise that right, you are being unkind to yourself. Be kind to yourself, before you extend the kindness to others.

1. Don't Bother about What Others Will Think

Often, a need to agree to unreasonable requests comes from a need for 'approval' from others. We are afraid that we will be disliked if we say no. We're worried about what others will think of us. This is especially so among teens and people in their twenties. But consider this: if someone's approval of you is dependent on your saying yes to every single thing they ask of you, then you don't need them in your life. They are clearly using you.

As we get older, we grow and realize this. We learn to be comfortable with who we are. I will hit my fifties soon, and I am more confident than I ever was in my twenties. I am not worried about other people's opinions of me. My friends who are older tell me it only gets better. We stop caring about other people's opinions of us.

I have learnt that no matter how nice you are and how sincere your intentions are, people will have their own opinions about your actions—and not always positive ones. If I had known this in my twenties, I would have been much more assertive.

2. Don't Give an Answer Straight Away

When I first started practising assertiveness, one of the things I learnt to do was stall for time. I fought my instinct to immediately say yes. I consciously began saying, 'I need some time to think about it; let me get back to you on this.' I discovered this was a great way to escape saying yes. Most people don't expect an immediate answer. They are understanding when we say that we need time. I use this especially when people call me up out of the blue and ask for a favour.

Whenever you are asked to do something that you don't want to do, the best option is to stall for time.

Principle 2: Prioritizing Your Well-being Does Not Make You Selfish

1. Consider Whether You Are Being Used

Once you have the time to take a decision, think about how many requests this person has made in the past, and whether you mind doing it for them. Be objective about how they treat you. Do they only call you up for favours? If the tables were turned, would they do the same for you? After considering all the factors, decide whether you want to say yes or no.

Please remember that whenever we give someone our time, we are giving them a piece of our life we will never get back. So before you do, ask yourself if they are worth your time.

2. Don't Justify Yourself

We often feel guilty or selfish or overly worried when we say no. If you decide to say no, don't be apologetic. Instead, practise saying these phrases:

- It doesn't work for me right now.
- It does sound lovely, but I will have to pass. Perhaps another time?
- I'm really swamped at the moment, and I simply can't.
- Thank you for thinking of me, but I just can't at the moment.
- I will not be able to make it. But thank you for asking.
- I have a lot going on right now.

By using these phrases, you are putting yourself first and not allowing others to take advantage of you. It's a form of self-care/self-love.

3. Become Your Own Cheerleader

Humans are inclined to look for validation, but it is important to stop craving other people's approval for everything that we do. If we keep attempting to please others at our own expense, we will end up putting ourselves last and become increasingly unhappy.

Often, we are very harsh on ourselves. By treating ourselves the way we would treat a valued friend, we become more forgiving and kinder towards ourselves. A friend of mine has a rule wherein she watches herself talk and asks herself if it is something that she will say to a friend. If the answer is no, she isn't allowed to say it to herself.

Practise prioritizing yourself. It is important to embrace your authentic self and tell yourself that you are worthy of love and kindness. You don't need validation from the outside world. Once you learn to accept and love yourself, you will become content and stop craving external validation. Subsequently, the need to please others will go away. Learning to say no requires practice and is a constant process. Putting yourself first is not being selfish. Work on cultivating the habit of self-love. Don't be afraid of being judged. Since it is a learnt practice, you will have to keep at it. Progress may be slow, but as long as you are aware, you will eventually get there! It gets easier as you grow older and become surer of who you are.

Magic Mindset for Saying No

Principle 1: You Have the Right to Say No
Principle 2: Prioritizing Your Well-being Does Not Make You Selfish

Say No to Unreasonable Requests

1. Don't Bother about What Others Will Think
2. Don't Give an Answer Straight Away
3. Consider Whether You Are Being Used
4. Don't Justify Yourself
5. Become Your Own Cheerleader

14

The Magic Mindset for Social Media

People have to share everything they do these days, from meals, to nights out, to selfies of themselves half naked in a mirror. The borders between public and private are dissolving.

—Bernardine Evaristo

I GREW UP IN THE PRE-INTERNET AND PRE-TELEVISION ERA. We first got a television only when I was fourteen or so. Hence most of my childhood was television free. By the time the internet became accessible and affordable, I was already a mother with a young baby. The first connections that we had were 'dial-up' connections. Anyone from the nineties would remember the whirring noises while the modem was dialling the servers. Sometimes, it would connect only after several attempts. There were no laptops, only unwieldy desktops—the 386 and 486. I have always been fascinated with technology, and when I first heard the term 'information super-highway', I was certain I wanted to cruise, despite the speed of the connection (compared to what we have today) being so slow.

Though things are so different now, I still cannot get over how much technology has advanced and how fortunate I am to be living in this era. Today, I have two internet connections from two different service providers, one of which offers an astonishing speed of 300 Mbps; if one is down, the other acts as a backup and we are effectively always connected. I have a good social media presence on almost all the major platforms—Twitter, Instagram, Facebook. I was even on TikTok until it was banned in India. I genuinely enjoy sharing things on social media, and I am excited about new features. Many of my childhood friends barely use it, as it wasn't a part of our lives. But if we want to keep up with the times, social media is something we can't avoid.

For most people between the ages of fourteen and thirty-five, it is a huge part of their life. Even older folks find it hard to stay away from social media and the messaging apps once they have got a taste of it. After all, it is convenient, quick and easy; with a few clicks, you get access to vast amounts of information.

But like everything else in the world, it does have down sides too. Numerous studies published in scientific journals[13] have linked the excessive use of social media to depression, anxiety, poor sleep and a feeling of unworthiness. Even though

---

13 Melissa Hunt, Rachel Marx, Courtney Lipson, Jordyn Young, *Journal of Social and Clinical Psychology*.

social media is supposed to help us connect with our friends and loved ones, it ironically leads to loneliness and sadness. The reason? We *compare* our lives to our friends' lives, or at least the version they post on social media. The more time we spend on social media, the more isolated we end up feeling. We scroll through hundreds of photos, and we feel our lives are lacking. 'FOMO' or the *fear of missing out* is very real.

A few years back, when I was working on my third book, I discovered that all the ladies in my residential building had gone out for a movie, and they hadn't invited me. I remember feeling really upset about it, and I told my husband. He asked me whether going for a movie was important or focusing on my book. That helped me, and I got over the incident quickly.

The thing to note, though, is that despite being a busy adult, with two children and a home to take care of, I still felt left out over something minor. I can only imagine the impact such a thing would have on young, susceptible minds who have grown up on social media. Many young people write to me asking me to give a shout-out to their accounts so that their friends are impressed. Social media is a world of 'showing off', with people only revealing the 'perfect' side of their lives.

Avoiding social media altogether is probably not possible in today's times. But how do we use it to our advantage? How can we stop it from affecting us negatively?

Principle 1: Remember that Social Media Is a Small Part of Real Life

These days, almost everything we experience is shared online. Twitter, Instagram or Facebook mimic each other, encouraging their users to share 'stories' or 'fleets', which vanish in twenty-four hours. The temptation is hard to resist. We click pictures of the food we eat, jewellery we liked, a quote we came across, or any thought that occurs to us. We rarely pause and think about what we share. After all, it vanishes in twenty-four hours, and there's always the delete button.

1. Real Life Is Not Online

If we follow a lot of people, we have hundreds of these random stories to browse through. Often, they are entertaining and give us a small burst of joy. The more we browse, the more distracted we are. The content is fun, and we get hooked very quickly. But we must remember that if we constantly go through other people's stories, we will invariably end up comparing. The more 'fun stuff' we see, the duller our own life seems in comparison. One friend has made a delicious looking tiramisu, another has drawn a stunning portrait, yet another has shared his workout stories and so on.

Ask yourself if you are truly interested in what your friends are up to every day. If we follow fifty people, and they all post just three stories, we have gone through 150 fifteen-second stories. We have spent 2,250 seconds just browsing. That's thirty-seven minutes of our time! What have we gained from these thirty-seven minutes? Make conscious choices when it comes to what you spend time on. Be aware of how it makes you feel at the end of it. If it doesn't make you feel good, stop!

2. Things Are Highly Styled for Social Media

A few weeks back, I was doing an online course on interior design from a renowned interior stylist. She was demonstrating the various ways in which she would style a room. She said that if it was for Instagram, she would add a ton of extra accessories, so it would look great in the pictures. But if it's a space that will be lived in and used, then she wouldn't recommend adding those things.

Most of the content we see on Instagram or other social media is like that. It is curated specifically to induce an emotion or a mood. We only see bits of people's lives—tiny aspects that show off the best parts. When we see a photo and read the caption, we don't think much about what goes on behind the scenes. Pictures only capture a moment. But there might be a whole story we are unaware of. When people post on Instagram, they do it mostly to make themselves feel good. The bit that they share might be genuine, but their life is not as picture-perfect as their posts have us believe. Nobody's life is. They might have problems that are worse than ours. They might be going through anxiety or depression. They may have a parent who is dying. We can never know the full story from a few posts.

Most influencers admit that the content they share is carefully curated. When it comes to Instagram and other social media, seeing is not believing!

Principle 2: Audit Time Spent and Accounts Followed on Social Media

To use social media with a magic mindset, where it leaves us feeling good and energized, here are a few things that we can do.

1. Follow a Limited Number of Accounts

If you check my Instagram account, you will see that I follow less than ten people. When I spoke to young adults, they told me following and unfollowing someone is an important thing for them. One couldn't abruptly 'unfollow' someone; it was considered rude. I was told that if they did that, the person whom they unfollowed would message them and ask them about it. Even if unfollowing is not an option, we can go to the settings and mute all the accounts we truly do not want to know about.

Think about it. *How much do you really care whether an acquaintance went to Spain or Cambodia for a holiday, or what they are up to currently?* If we do want to know, we can search for their accounts whenever we want to and check their posts.

Following someone gives them a permanent spot on our minds. It is akin to leaving the front door wide open and letting anyone wander in.

As a writer, my mind is my greatest asset. I have to be very careful who I let inside. This goes for non-writers too. If we keep scrolling through other people's feeds, we are giving them an open invitation to occupy our precious mind-space. *Don't!* Take control of who you let in, and either unfollow or mute. Those buttons are there for a reason. Use them.

2. Check What You Get from It

Every now and then, we must check what we get from the accounts we do follow. I have an art account as well as a regular account. On my art account, all the accounts I follow are those whose art styles I absolutely love. The moment I go through them, I am inspired. It makes me want to create art. I carefully scrutinize the accounts and choose ones that have a style that fills me with awe. I also make it a point to comment on posts I particularly loved. I gain a lot from following these accounts; they help me fill up my creative well.

On my regular account, I follow only family and a couple of inspirational fitness accounts, since fitness is one of my main interests. Again, the fitness accounts I follow are those that I have personally connected with and from which I get motivated to work out. There are many fitness accounts out there, but many set impossible standards. They might have put in the hard work for what they have achieved, but if it constantly makes us feel that we aren't good enough, we don't need to follow them. I am always pruning the list of people I follow. Sometimes, the public figures we follow deviate from their typical content. At times, we might outgrow the content they create. They change or we might change. If the accounts we follow start posting things that no longer resonate with us, we must not hesitate to unfollow.

Do a periodic audit of the accounts that you engage with and be conscious that you are allowing them into your mind, thereby giving them permission to influence your mood and well-being. So be very picky.

3. Go on Detoxes

Several young people I know go on social media detoxes from time to time. They say they are tired of being 'hooked to the phone' all the time. They deactivate their social media accounts for about a week, and some have gone up to thirty days.

They all report that their attention span increased, their anxiety decreased and the time at their disposal increased. They said the pressure to 'create posts' was gone and they didn't have to spend time 'liking' other people's posts and getting involved in the 'drama'.

Most of them reported feeling more peaceful, and they also read more. We're all enmeshed in this digital world, and we all like to feel loved, accepted and validated—even if it comes from complete strangers.

Try taking a detox from social media and see how you feel.

As long as we have control over how we use social media, it can be a great tool. If we use it to follow accounts that give us joy, that teach us something or inspire us, then it is all good. But often, we do not know where to stop.

If this has happened to you, step back and try the steps above. You're likely to feel happier once you get over the initial discomfort of suddenly being disconnected. You don't need social media to connect with real friends—you would pick up the phone and make a call!

Magic Mindset for Social Media

Principle 1: Remember that Social Media Is a Small Part of Real Life
Principle 2: Audit Time Spent and Accounts Followed On Social Media

Remember:

1. Real Life Is Not Online
2. Things Are Highly Styled for Social Media

Practice:

1. Follow a Limited Number of Accounts
2. Check What You Get from It
3. Go on Detoxes

PART 4

*Fun with the Magic Mindset!
A 14-Day Activity Challenge
to Help You Start
Your Journey into the Magic
Mindset*

PART 1

15
The 14-Day Challenge

Kindness in words creates confidence. Kindness in thinking creates profoundness. Kindness in giving creates love.

—Lao Tzu

THE ONLY WAY TO PRACTICE THE MAGIC MINDSET IS TO actually do it! Perhaps you are ready to make a change in your thinking, but you don't know where to start. Perhaps you're cocooned in lethargy and simply cannot bring yourself to do anything or perhaps you are in a place where nothing excites you any more.

If you are in a place where you are not happy, are fed up with your career, tired of life and generally dissatisfied with everything going on around you, *it is time to take charge*. It may not be possible to change your situation overnight, but you can definitely take tiny steps to change your mindset.

Ready for some fun challenges to help you into the magic mindset?

I've put together a fourteen-day activity plan. These might seem like 'silly activities' or even absurd, because you have never done anything like it. The 'logical' part of your brain might tell you, 'Doing these activities will not change my situation.' Or, 'How is this going to help me?'

Please discard all these thoughts. Just try these activities. You have nothing to lose! Make a resolution to follow them diligently. Please don't expect to feel happy instantly, as soon as you do one of these activities (although that may happen too!). Sometimes, you may not feel anything after you do it. But it is important to do all the tasks listed here.

The Rules:

1. You can start whenever you like.
2. Once you begin, please don't stop midway.
3. If you miss a day, you can choose from any of the activities you have completed till that date and repeat one of them, before you proceed to the next activity.

For added fun, share the Magic Mindset Challenge with a friend.

Changing a mindset is a slow process. It requires conscious and constant effort. The tasks I have listed here are tiny steps in that direction, to give you a nudge, especially if you have fallen into a set pattern. Every activity that you do gets added to the 'Magic Mindset Bank'. By doing these tasks, you are making tiny deposits of happiness.

Once you set a date to start the challenge, it is important to stick to it. I have elaborated on the way that you can carry out the activity. I have also included simpler options. You can make your own modifications to anything I suggest. These are only guidelines.

You will not require more than thirty minutes a day to do the activities mentioned. Some of them may not even take that long. Use the chart at the end of the chapter to record the date when you do an activity, as well as how you feel immediately after. For the first week, the focus is on YOU. You're going to be doing all these things that will make you feel good about yourself.

Week 1

Day 1: Simple Massage for Tired Feet

Things needed: coconut oil, olive oil, mustard oil, a large towel, an old pair of slippers

Take a bowl and add 3 tablespoons of mustard oil, 3 tablespoons of olive oil and 3 tablespoons of coconut oil. Mix well with a spoon. Keep the pair of old 'Hawaii *chappals*' next to you before you begin the activity. Also spread a large towel on the floor. You could omit the towel, but I have discovered it is smarter to use one, because it makes things easier and avoids getting oil on the floor.

Sit in the middle of the towel. If you have difficulty sitting on the floor, use a small bathroom stool. Take your left foot and rest it gently on your right thigh. Now, apply the oil mixture to the sole of your foot. Begin with the toes and massage each toe in a circular motion. Vary the pressure. You can use your knuckles for extra pressure.

Next, massage the heel in a circular motion. Use both your hands to do this. Feel all the nerves that end at your foot. You are stimulating the blood flow to the nerve by massaging it. Gently pull the toes apart. Massage between the toes. Encircle your toes by slipping your fingers in between the toes and grasp them. Now gently rotate them. Also massage your ankles. Repeat the process on the other foot. You could play your favourite songs and give yourself a foot massage for the duration of the song, say, two songs for each foot.

That's it! Your activity for Day 1 is done. You will feel a lot lighter after you do this. I offered to do this for both my children, and they loved it as well. They later did it for me. What joy and relaxation this simple activity brought!

Note: Please be careful when you wear your old slippers and walk to the bathroom to wash off the oil. The first time I tried this activity, I was so delighted, it felt like I was 'walking on air'.

Day 2: Organize Your Desk/Wardrobe

Choose either your desk or your wardrobe (whichever you haven't tidied for a while). Take out every single item. This is a technique Marie Kondo uses. I am a huge fan of the Konmari method of tidying and have used her methods to change the way I store and organize things.[14]

---

14 *The Life-Changing Magic of Tidying Up* is indeed a book that changed my life.

When I first followed this method, I discovered that I had a lot of expensive dresses I had bought many years ago. My sense of personal style had changed since then. While those dresses were expensive, I knew I would no longer wear them. I gave them away and felt much lighter.

If you have chosen to tidy your wardrobe, take out every item that you haven't worn in the last six months. Think about whether you really want to hold on to them. They might be expensive items or sentimental items. You might be holding on to them for 'when you lose weight'. They might have been items that were useful to you at one point in your life, but if they no longer fit or if you do not like the way you look in them, it is time to let them go, no matter how expensive they are. Marie Kondo suggests 'thanking the item' and sending it on its way.

There might be items in your wardrobe that need a little mending. A button might have come off or there might be a small tear you intended getting around to but put off. Fixing it would make it wearable, but you kept procrastinating. If so, this is the time to fix it. Finally, fold the clothes that you decide to keep and arrange them back into the wardrobe.

That's it! Your task for Day 2 is complete. Share before and after pictures if you want to! Use the hashtag #themagicmindset so I can find it on social media.

Note: If you have a very large wardrobe and have neglected it for a long period of time, consider doing just one shelf. Whenever I tidy my wardrobe, I find it tiresome to do the whole thing in a single day, so I spread it over a few days, targeting one shelf a day.

Day 3: Make a Change in Your Room

Our living spaces have great influence on our mood and how we feel. Neuroscientists and psychologists affirm that there are specialized cells in the hippocampal regions of our brain that react to the design and colours used in the spaces we occupy. Think of all the places you have lived in and think of the way they made you feel. What was the place like? Was it bright and airy? Was it tidy? Did it have many interesting objects? What did the place mean to you?

The colours that surround us, the furnishings we use, the way we arrange our room—all of it matters. Making a change in the interiors of a room changes the 'energy flow'. We don't need to have expensive interiors and change the colour of the walls or do extreme makeovers to feel happier. We can achieve the same by making a small change.

A friend of mine was once on a tight budget for the curtains in her bedroom. She used her mother's old sarees and got her local tailor to make unique looking beautiful ethnic drapes. She also used locally available straw mats, got some inexpensive cushions, and made a low seating. With a budget of less than two thousand rupees she transformed her bedroom completely. In fact, you don't even have to spend money to make a change in your room.

Look around your room and think of what you want to change. It could be as simple as changing the bedsheets to a clean, colour-coordinated set. Maybe you can buy inexpensive fairy lights and add that to your room. Perhaps you can change the position of the furniture. You could get a glass covering added to your desk and use the part under the glass to display your goals or your favourite pictures. Maybe you could get some fresh flowers every day. The change you make could be as simple as tidying the room, cleaning everything thoroughly, and getting rid of the things that are no longer useful. Unleash your creative imagination and make a change in your living space right away!

Your task for Day 3 is now complete! You can now relax with your favourite beverage in your freshly made room. Enjoy!

Day 4: Try a New Recipe

Trying something new increases our creative capacity. Every time we put ourselves in a situation we have not encountered before, we are giving some 'new work' to our brains. In response, the neurons will fire, assimilating the information needed to perform the new task, making calculations and then sending out the signals to act in a certain manner.

When both my children were living abroad while attending college, they learnt to cook. After eating out for most of their meals, they found cooking a refreshing experience. Both said they had no idea it was this easy and that they could save such a lot of money by learning how to cook. Both make interesting dishes now—things that they taught themselves. For my husband's birthday, I gifted him an exclusive baking workshop (because he loves cakes). He had always made cakes using the ready-mix packets available in stores. Learning to make cakes from scratch was an activity he tremendously enjoyed.

If you have been cooking for a long time and are used to similar kinds of food, try something completely new. Perhaps you can try to cook a Mexican dish or Arabian dish. By trying to do something new, you are stimulating not only your brain but also your tastebuds.

Pick an easy recipe with ingredients that you can easily source. If you have never cooked before, try making a simple dish—perhaps one that your mother cooks. Ask her for the instructions.

Your task for Day 4 is now complete! Enjoy what you made, and make sure that you put in a little effort in presentation as well.

Day 5: Detox from Social Media

Social media can be stimulating and inspiring. We like to unwind by looking at great pictures on Pinterest or Instagram. We like to see what our favourite blogger or Instagrammer is posting. We idly browse through other people's stories and photos. We read up stuff that interests us. We look for memes that make us laugh. A funny video catches our attention, and even before we realize it, an hour has gone by! The internet is a black hole that sucks up our time without us even realizing it.

A few years back, I discovered the power of turning off my phone. I wanted to read more than I was currently reading and had a reading goal of about four to five books a month. I discovered that my phone was the main culprit in consuming my time. I lived in a duplex house, and whenever it was my reading time, I would leave my phone on silent mode in my bedroom downstairs and head upstairs to read. I had a hammock in my garden, and it was relaxing to read in my hammock, with no interference or temptation to check the phone every fifteen minutes.

Today, turn off your phone for four to six hours during the day. Choose a time when you are usually browsing online and lock the phone away. No matter how strong the temptation is, do not turn it back on. If you don't trust yourself, give your phone to a family member or a friend. Most people find this activity hard, because we are so hooked to the phone that we feel 'something amiss' if we aren't connected all the time. Facebook and YouTube videos are designed in such a way that even before we finish watching the current video, another one pops up.

By making a choice to distance yourself from your phone for a few hours, you are empowering yourself to make healthier and more conscious decisions. You will also suddenly discover 'extra time' in your day, since the time spent on social media is often unaccounted for. You can use this time that you have 'freed up' for other activities that give you joy.

That's it! Your task for Day 5 is now complete.

Day 6: Dress Well

At the time of writing this, many of us had been working from home for several months. In response to the constraints brought on by the pandemic, companies cut down their office spaces, 'work from home' for at least half the week becoming the new normal.

In such a time, we don't feel a need or desire to 'dress up'. We're happy to lounge in our pyjamas and take our work calls or attend online classes from our beds. However, at times like these, it is even more important to dress well! Psychologists say that it has a direct effect on our mood, confidence and general approach to life. We don't even need science to back this up; when we dress well and are well-groomed, our mood improves.

So today, your task is to dress up like you are going on a date. Groom yourself. Wear a nice perfume. Do everything that makes you feel good. If you feel like it, set up your camera on self-timer and click a few pictures. (If you post them on social media, use #TheMagicMindset so I can find them.)

That's it! Your task for Day 6 is done.

Day 7: Gift Yourself Something

When was the last time you bought yourself a gift? Well, consider this the right occasion. It's time for a new gift, and you definitely deserve a good one.

Today, your task is to gift yourself something that will make you happy. If you have young kids, it could even be some alone time, with your favourite beverage, reading a book. When my children were little, I remember how pressed I was for time. I couldn't even shower in peace without one of the two knocking on the door, yelling, 'Mummy!'

It could be an online class you've been wanting to do. It could be new headphones you have been meaning to buy, but which you keep putting off, as your old ones are perfectly functional. Recently, I enrolled in a class by an artist whose work I greatly admire. I look forward to filling up my sketchbook with whatever I learnt in the class.

Today is the day to splurge on yourself. Gift yourself something nice. That's it! Your task for Day 7 is now done!

Record Your Progress

Day	Date	Task	How I felt after I completed it
1.		Massage Your Feet	
2.		Organize Desk/Wardrobe	
3.		Make a Change in Your Room	
4.		Try a New Recipe	
5.		Detox from Social Media	
6.		Dress Well	
7.		Gift Yourself Something	

Week 2

If you have completed all the tasks for Week 1, congratulations! You've graduated to Week 2. If you haven't completed a task, please go back and complete it. It is important to do the tasks in Week 1 because it prepares you for Week 2, which is all about making others feel good. We can do that only if we feel good ourselves. We need our own cups to be full before we can fill the cups of others.

Day 1: Smile and Greet

In 2017, Jehangir Art Gallery, a premier art space in Mumbai, hosted an unusual photography exhibition called 'So I Asked Them to Smile'. It featured the work of Jay Weinstein, an Australian-born travel guide and photographer, who specializes in India. Jay had photographed random strangers from several countries. In this exhibition, paired photos were displayed—the first photo of the person without a smile, and the second one of them smiling. The visual impact is stunning.

Jay says that in 2013, he was in Bikaner, working on a photography project. It was dusk, and he was wandering around the Junagarh fort. He was busy clicking pictures and found himself passing the markets, the railway station and the streets. Night fell, and he was about to put away his camera when he noticed a man directly in front of him. The man had a deep green skull cap, a wispy beard and a narrow face. Jay wanted to photograph him, but he hesitated as the man looked stern with a stony expression in his eyes. Jay was intimidated, so he instead began photographing other things. Suddenly, the man called out to him, asking him to take his picture too. Jay asked him to smile, and he did. In that instant, the person was transformed. His face had warmth and his eyes twinkled with humour. He no longer looked intimidating. Jay decided in that moment that he would document the effect of a smile on a stranger's face. Jay says his goal is to demonstrate how we view a stranger, and how our assumptions change when they smile.

Today's task is inspired from Jay's project. Go for a walk and call out a cheery 'good morning' or 'good evening' to three people who cross your path. They can be strangers or people known to you. Gift them a genuine smile. If they smile back, observe how their face transforms. If they don't smile, that's okay too.

Spread kindness and cheer. If you've never done this before, you might find it hard to do so. Make an effort to just smile at one person and greet them. Notice how different you feel: when we smile, despite how we feel inside, our brains release 'feel-good' endorphins.

That's it! Your task for Day 1 of Week 2 is done!

Day 2: Surprise Someone with Flowers or a Gift

A few weeks back, I received a beautiful package in the mail. It contained a lovely handmade box with some incense made in Auroville, a gorgeous little stone bracelet, some incense cones and a book written by the person who sent it. It was aesthetically gift-wrapped, and I was delighted to receive such a thoughtful gift hamper. It brightened my day. I, too, have sent books as gifts to many of my friends. I have even gifted plants; one time, I made a miniature garden and gifted it to my neighbour. There was no 'special occasion' to do so.

When we give a gift to somebody, we make their day special. Today, your task is to brighten someone's day. Think about what they would really like. Then gift it to them!

That's it. Your task for Day 2 of Week 2 is complete.

Day 3: Share an Inspiring Story

Today, look up an inspiring story on the internet. It could be a rags-to-riches story or just a story about an unsung hero. There are many sites such as The Better India that focus only on positive stories.

Read a few, and when you come across something or someone truly inspirational, share it! You could share it with a friend or a family member, or you could tweet a link on social media. (If you want me to see it, please use the hashtag #TheMagicMindset.) Describe what you admire and like about the story. In case you know a real-life hero who is underappreciated, you can share their story too.

When we share positive and uplifting stories, we are spreading hope and positivity. Be an ambassador of hope today!

That's it! Your task for Day 3 of Week 2 is done.

Day 4: Call a Senior Citizen or a Friend

Set aside some time in your day and make a phone call to a senior citizen in your life. It could be your aunt, your parents or simply a friend. Talk to them, enquire about what they are doing and listen to them. In case you have no senior citizens in your life, simply call someone whom you have been meaning to call for a long time. Do not put it off.

Research shows that loneliness is on the rise.[15] We all live in a connected world, but we're also cocooned in our own thoughts, fears and anxieties. Sometimes, we get so busy with our careers that we forget to keep in touch with close friends and even family. Connecting with others not only makes them feel loved, wanted and cared for, but also helps us. Social scientists point out that the genuine connections we form are huge mood boosters.

Today, pick up the phone and have a long, nice chat with someone you have been neglecting for a while. You should have a genuine connection with this person.

That's it! Your task for Day 4, Week 2 is done.

---

15 *The Hindu*, 13 May 2019 and the Cigna Loneliness Index, 2020.

Day 5: Write a Kind Message or Note

Think about anyone you know or a co-worker you have observed. Write a kind note to them, paying them a compliment. Ensure that what you say is genuine, kind and sincere. You could compliment them on something you have noticed. Perhaps they have a great sense of style or they are kind to everyone or you like how cheerful they are.

Just imagine their joy and surprise when they read it.

That's it! Your task for Day 5, Week 2 is done.

Day 6: Say Only Positive Things

Our minds chatter endlessly to us. Today is the day when you must pay attention and be aware of what your mind says. Most humans tend to think negatively. Researchers tell us that 80 per cent of our thoughts are negative![16]

Today, your task is to be aware of all the thoughts that are flooding your mind, notice the patterns and squish them or replace them with another thought that phrases the same sentiment positively. For every negative thought that comes into your head, immediately think about three positives. Try to think about what could be positive about the situation and repeat that to yourself.

Also, anything you say today has to be kind and positive. Whether it is on social media or to your family members, say only kind things—just for today.

That's it! Your task for Day 6 of Week 2 is done.

---

[16] National Science Foundation study.

Day 7: Cook a Meal for a Homeless Person

When we give without expecting anything in return, we feel joy. Altruistic behaviour causes an endorphin rush. Narayanan Krishnan is a real-life hero and a huge inspiration for many. He was an award-winning chef at a five-star hotel and was shortlisted for an elite job in Switzerland. He was scheduled to leave the country, but an incident he witnessed in his hometown deeply disturbed him. He saw an old person eating faecal waste due to hunger. Krishnan approached a nearby hotel and bought idlis for the man. He says he has never seen someone eating so fast, with tears of gratitude streaming down his face. It was a moment that changed Krishnan. He quit his job and decided to feed the homeless with his savings. His parents and family thought he had gone mad, but Krishnan was certain of what he wanted to do.

Today, he has established a trust that feeds and houses lakhs of destitute people. The trust is supported by many corporate organizations that want to support the good work Krishnan is doing. In 2010, Krishnan was recognized as one of the world's top ten heroes by CNN.

While we can't replicate what Krishnan has done, we can do a small bit. Today, cook a meal for a homeless person. If you get most of your meals from outside, just buy bread and butter and make a simple sandwich. Pack the meal well. Go out and look for a homeless person. In India, sadly, we find aged people who beg for money at almost every traffic signal. You can also find people outside places of worship. Hand them a hot meal.

That's it! Your task for Day 7 of Week 2 is complete.

Record Your Progress

Day	Date	Task	How I felt after I completed it
1.		Smile and Greet	
2.		Surprise Someone with a Gift or Flowers	
3.		Share an Inspiring Story	
4.		Call a Senior Citizen or a Friend	
5.		Leave an Anonymous Kind Note	
6.		Say Only Positive Things	
7.		Cook a Meal for a Homeless Person	

***

I hope you enjoyed performing these little acts and that they gave you something to look forward to each day. The tips and activities that I have shared here will help you in your journey towards a magic mindset, which will help you take care of yourself better. If you did do these activities, please post it publicly to inspire others as well. Use the hashtag #TheMagicMindset.

Life is truly beautiful. We only have to focus on what is right. And no matter what your situation is, it WILL change. Everything we are going through is just another step forward on the long journey called life. Life has taught me that we all will have at least a few problems at any given point in our lives. If we focus on the hopelessness of the situation, it makes us miserable. All we can do is take it one day at a time and take tiny steps to make our present realities a little bit better.

The true magic in the 'magic mindset' happens when we learn to let go of the things we cannot control and be deeply grateful for the things we have already been blessed with. I hope this book helps you discover that there is magic within all of us. We can lead more fulfilling, happier and peaceful lives when we accept this magic—focusing on the abundance and joy we have and creating happy memories with the people we value.

Acknowledgements

To my father, K.V.J. Kamath, for all that he taught me and to my mother, Priya Kamath, for being my strength.

To my wonderful editor, Swati Daftuar, for believing so much in the book, and making it so much better. It's such a joy to work with someone whose vision syncs with yours. Her ability to completely get what I am trying to communicate astounds me, each time.

To the superb team at Harper Collins—Ananth Padmanabhan, Diya Kar, Shabnam Srivatsava, Rahul Dixit.

To the cover designer, Saurav Das, for a brilliant cover and layout of the book.

To my technical support team Pranav Shah who is super responsive.

To my three—Atul, Purvi and Satish for always being my biggest cheerleaders.

To my closest friends who I am in touch with on a regular basis—you know who you are!

To all my lovely readers who tell me how much my words mean to them, and how it makes their lives better. I am honoured that you choose to share bits of your life with me, it means so much and I am overwhelmed by your support and your trust in me.

About the Author

Preeti Shenoy, among the highest selling authors in India, is on the Forbes longlist of the most influential celebrities in India. Her books include *When Love Came Calling, Wake Up Life is Calling, Life Is What You Make It, The Rule Breakers, A Hundred Little Flames, It's All in the Planets, Why We Love the Way We Do, The Secret Wish List, The One You Cannot Have* and many others. Her work has been translated into many Indian languages. Preeti is also a motivational speaker, and has given talks at many premier educational institutions and corporate organizations like KPMG, ISRO, Infosys and Accenture, among others. An avid fitness enthusiast, she is also an artist specialising in portraiture and illustrated journalling.